Marine de Chefdebien
Pascal Clerc

Les infections à répétition de l'enfant

Marine de Chefdebien
Pascal Clerc

Les infections à répétition de l'enfant

Typologie de 1014 enfants atteints de pathologies infectieuses aiguës, nés entre 1999 et 2001, suivis pendant 10 ans

Presses Académiques Francophones

Impressum / Mentions légales
Bibliografische Information der Deutschen Nationalbibliothek: Die Deutsche Nationalbibliothek verzeichnet diese Publikation in der Deutschen Nationalbibliografie; detaillierte bibliografische Daten sind im Internet über http://dnb.d-nb.de abrufbar.
Alle in diesem Buch genannten Marken und Produktnamen unterliegen warenzeichen-, marken- oder patentrechtlichem Schutz bzw. sind Warenzeichen oder eingetragene Warenzeichen der jeweiligen Inhaber. Die Wiedergabe von Marken, Produktnamen, Gebrauchsnamen, Handelsnamen, Warenbezeichnungen u.s.w. in diesem Werk berechtigt auch ohne besondere Kennzeichnung nicht zu der Annahme, dass solche Namen im Sinne der Warenzeichen- und Markenschutzgesetzgebung als frei zu betrachten wären und daher von jedermann benutzt werden dürften.

Information bibliographique publiée par la Deutsche Nationalbibliothek: La Deutsche Nationalbibliothek inscrit cette publication à la Deutsche Nationalbibliografie; des données bibliographiques détaillées sont disponibles sur internet à l'adresse http://dnb.d-nb.de.
Toutes marques et noms de produits mentionnés dans ce livre demeurent sous la protection des marques, des marques déposées et des brevets, et sont des marques ou des marques déposées de leurs détenteurs respectifs. L'utilisation des marques, noms de produits, noms communs, noms commerciaux, descriptions de produits, etc., même sans qu'ils soient mentionnés de façon particulière dans ce livre ne signifie en aucune façon que ces noms peuvent être utilisés sans restriction à l'égard de la législation pour la protection des marques et des marques déposées et pourraient donc être utilisés par quiconque.

Coverbild / Photo de couverture: www.ingimage.com

Verlag / Editeur:
Presses Académiques Francophones
ist ein Imprint der / est une marque déposée de
OmniScriptum GmbH & Co. KG
Heinrich-Böcking-Str. 6-8, 66121 Saarbrücken, Deutschland / Allemagne
Email: info@presses-academiques.com

Herstellung: siehe letzte Seite /
Impression: voir la dernière page
ISBN: 978-3-8416-3430-6

Zugl. / Agréé par: Versailles, Université de Versailles Saint Quentin en Yvelines, 2013

Copyright / Droit d'auteur © 2015 OmniScriptum GmbH & Co. KG
Alle Rechte vorbehalten. / Tous droits réservés. Saarbrücken 2015

REMERCIEMENTS :

Au Docteur Pascal CLERC,
Un immense merci de m'avoir accompagnée, coachée et soutenue durant la rédaction de cet ouvrage. Merci également de m'avoir aidée à trouver ce sujet si passionnant, et du temps précieux que tu m'as accordé.

Au Docteur Philippe BOISNAULT,
Merci pour ton aide précieuse concernant les données de la base de l'OMG, sans lesquelles cet ouvrage n'aurait pu voir le jour.

Au Docteur Olivier SAINT LARY,
Merci pour ces trois années d'internat en tant que tuteur, pendant lesquelles tu as su me prêter une oreille attentive et me donner des conseils toujours avisés.

A Antonin,
Merci pour ton amour si précieux, ton soutien tout au long de nos études et pour l'immense bonheur que tu m'offres en vivant chaque jour à mes côtés.
Merci également pour le regard bienveillant que tu as toujours porté sur mes choix professionnels, et pour m'avoir encouragée à aller toujours plus loin.

A mes parents,
Pour votre amour et votre soutien inébranlable. La confiance que vous avez mise en moi et la fierté que j'ai toujours lue dans vos yeux quel que soit mon parcours. Ma réussite vous revient en grande partie et je n'en serais pas là sans vous.

A ma famille,
Pour votre amour précieux et vos encouragements pendant ces longues années d'études. Merci d'avoir toujours cru en moi et de m'avoir soutenue comme vous l'avez fait.

A ma belle-famille,
Pour votre amour et votre soutien depuis le premier jour.

A mes amis, sans qui la vie ne serait pas aussi belle,

A mes co-internes avec qui j'ai partagé joies et galères d'internat.

A tous les médecins que j'ai eu la chance de côtoyer ou de croiser pendant mes études, ceux qui ont pris le temps de me former, et ceux qui m'ont marquée par leur humanité et leurs compétences mises au service du patient.

Table des matières

I. CONTEXTE : 5
II. OBJECTIFS : 17
III. MATERIEL ET MÉTHODE : 18
   A. TYPE D'ÉTUDE : 18
   B. Analyse bibliographique : 18
   C. Matériel : 20
      1. Observatoire de Médecine Générale (OMS) : 20
      2. Base d'étude et variables utilisées : 21
   D. Méthode: 23
IV. ANALYSE DESCRIPTIVE : 25
   A. Les patients : 25
   B. Les actes : 25
   C. Les résultats de consultation : 26
   D. Les Résultat de consultation infectieux : 27
      1. En fonction du sexe : 27
      2. En fonction du lieu d'habitation: 28
      3. En fonction de la classe d'âge : 30
      4. En fonction des trois résultats de consultation représentant les deux tiers des pathologies infectieuses : 34
      5. En fonction du caractère aigüe ou persistant des résultats de consultation infectieux : 37
      6. Répartition du nombre d'infections par quartile et par classes d'âge : .. 38
      7. Répartition des enfants en fonction du nombre d'infections totales : 39
      8. Nombre de résultats de consultation infectieux différents par enfants: 40
   E. Distribution des comorbidités : 42
   F. Médecin traitant : 44
      1. Généralités 44
      2. Lieu d'exercice : 45
   G. Synthèse : 46
V. TYPOLOGIE : 49
   A. Analyse en correspondances multiples : 49
   B. Classification ascendante hiérarchique : 51
VI. ANALYSE DES TRAITEMENTS PAR ANTIBIOTIQUES : 59
   A. Analyse descriptive 59
   B. Analyse par classes de la typologie : 60
      1. Par prescription d'antibiotiques : 60
      2. Par nombre de patients recevant des antibiotiques : 62
VII. CHOIX DE LA CLASSE PERMETTANT DE REPÉRER LES ENFANTS LES PLUS INFECTÉS : 65
VIII. DISCUSSION : 67

IX.	CONCLUSION :	74
X.	BIBLIOGRAPHIE :	75
XI.	ANNEXES :	82
A.	ANNEXE n°1 : L'observatoire de médecine générale :	82
	1. Objectifs de l'Observatoire de la MG :	82
	2. Définition du résultat de consultation :	82
	3. Dictionnaire des Résultats de Consultation :	83
	4. Correspondance CIM 10 :	83
B.	ANNEXE n°2 : Résultats de consultation :	85
C.	ANNEXE n°3 : Définitions des dix pathologies infectieuses sélectionnées selon le dictionnaire des résultats de consultation :	92
	1. ANGINE (AMYGDALITE - PHARYNGITE)	92
	2. BRONCHITE AIGUË	93
	3. DIARRHEE NAUSEE VOMISSEMENT	93
	4. ÉTAT MORBIDE AFÉBRILE	94
	5. ÉTAT FÉBRILE	95
	6. OTITE MOYENNE	96
	7. PNEUMOPATHIE AIGUE	97
	8. RHINOPHARYNGITE –RHUME	98
	9. SINUSITE	98
	10. TOUX	99

I. **CONTEXTE** :

Un des motifs de consultation le plus fréquent en pédiatrie de ville concerne les pathologies infectieuses. En effet, une étude réalisée par Élisabeth GRIOT en 1995, présente un état des lieux des principaux résultats de consultations des enfants auprès de leurs généralistes dans le cadre d'un réseau informatisé de médecins généralistes(1). Cette étude a révélé que 45,7% de l'activité du généraliste auprès des nourrissons (0-2 ans) était en rapport avec la pathologie infectieuse, représentée par les résultats de consultation[1] suivants : état fébrile, rhinopharyngite, otite moyenne aigue, état afébrile, rhume, bronchite aigue, angine, diarrhée et vomissements, conjonctivite et rhinite. De même, chez les jeunes enfants âgés de 2 à 10 ans, avec 52,9% de pathologies infectieuses puis 28,1% chez les grands enfants (10 à 15 ans).

Au cours de mes différents stages d'interne en ville et en pédiatrie, j'ai remarqué, qu'il y avait des enfants que l'on voyait beaucoup plus souvent que d'autres en consultation pour des infections récidivantes, et dont les parents s'inquiétaient de l'existence d'un éventuel déficit immunitaire à dépister. J'ai décidé de m'intéresser de plus près à ce groupe d'enfants présentant des infections dites « à répétition ». En effet, comme le souligne Malhaoui et coll., « la notion d'infections répétées est un motif fréquent d'inquiétude pour les parents. Il représente un nombre important de consultations auprès de pédiatres libéraux ou hospitaliers »(2) ainsi que des généralistes, en raison de leur contribution importante à la morbidité chez les enfants(3) et entrainent des conséquences non négligeables pour l'enfant, notamment en terme d'absentéisme scolaire, de répercussion sur la qualité de vie de l'enfant et de son entourage.

---

[1] Le résultat de consultation (RC) est l'ensemble des conclusions diagnostiques du médecin au terme de la séance, pondérées par une position diagnostique et un code suivi.

Une première recherche bibliographique avec les mots clefs «infection récurrente», ou « récidivante », ou « répétée », ou « à répétition » dans un contexte pédiatrique, donne 108 réponses. Tous les articles traitant du sujet sont cependant unanimes sur un point : il est normal de faire plusieurs infections respiratoires, en tous cas dans les premières années de vie(4). La plupart du temps, « *il s'agit d'infections des voies aériennes supérieures récurrentes (otite moyenne aiguë, rhinopharyngite, angine, laryngite) ou respiratoires basses (trachéite, bronchite, bronchiolite) chez un enfant sain dont le système immunitaire se développe normalement* »(2). Ainsi, « *six à dix épisodes de rhinopharyngites sont la règle dans les premières années de vie, le pic de fréquence se situant entre six et 18 mois* »(4)(5). Ces rhinopharyngites répétées doivent être considérées comme un « *phénomène normal chez un nourrisson qui construit ses défenses immunitaires dans un environnement où il rencontre des virus* »(6). De la même manière, « *il est considéré «normal» pour un enfant avant l'âge de 2-3 ans de présenter jusqu'à six à huit infections des voies respiratoires supérieures par année* »(7).

En revanche, les définitions d'infections « répétées / récidivantes / récurrentes » utilisées sont variables et dépendantes des études (3)(4)(6)(7)(8)(9)(10)(11)(12)(13)(14)(15)(16)(17)(18). En effet il y a quasiment autant de définitions que d'études : « *plus de 5 infections respiratoires chez les enfants de 2 à 5 ans et plus 3 infections respiratoires chez les enfants de 6 à 10 ans* »(3) ; « *les infections sont récidivantes à partir de 6 épisodes au cours d'une période de 8,5 mois* »(8)(9) ; « *au moins 6 infections respiratoires à la même période* »(10)(11) ; « *au moins trois épisodes infectieux par période de trois mois* »(12); « *au moins un des critères suivants doit être présent pour diagnostiquer une infections récurrentes des voies respiratoires: ≥ 6 infections respiratoires par an, dont au moins une infection respiratoire par mois impliquant le voies aériennes supérieures de septembre à avril; ou ≥ 3 infections respiratoires par an impliquant les voies respiratoires inférieures* »(3) ; « *otites récidivantes : trois épisodes en 6 mois ou quatre épisodes en 1 an* »(6)(13) ; « *l'otite aiguë moyenne récidivante peut être arbitrairement définie par la survenue d'au moins 3 épisodes d'OMA en moins de 6 mois, séparés chacun par un intervalle libre d'au moins 3 semaines* »(8); « *l'otite moyenne aiguë récurrente peut être définie comme six ou plusieurs épisodes d'otite moyenne aiguë pendant une période de 12 mois* »(18) « *infections des voies respiratoires inférieures récurrentes si : a). au moins deux épisodes de pneumonie (avec résolution intermédiaire à la radiographie) en un an, ou b). plus de trois épisodes, quel que soit le laps de temps écoulé* »(7) ; « *épisodes infectieux récidivants à partir de 6 épisodes au cours d'une période de 8,5 mois, toutefois ce nombre varie en fonction du type d'infections, ainsi, les otites sont considérées comme fréquentes à partir de 2 épisodes survenus au cours de la période* »(8).

Une mise au point parue en 2005(4), sur les bilans et traitements des infections respiratoires récidivantes, fait un état des lieux des différentes définitions des infections récidivantes par organe :

- « *Les définitions d'otites récidivantes les plus admises internationalement sont : trois épisodes en six mois ou quatre épisodes en un an. Pour l'ensemble du groupe, la définition de quatre en un an n'est pas assez discriminante, en particulier chez les jeunes enfants gardés en collectivité* »(14).

- « *Les définitions d'angines récidivantes admises internationalement sont sept ou plus en une année ou dix durant les deux à trois dernières années* »(15).

- « *Pour les rhinopharyngites, il ne semble pas exister de définition internationalement admise, mais pour l'ensemble du groupe, « plus de six épisodes de rhinopharyngites fébriles par an après l'âge de trois ans » semble acceptable* »(4).

- « *Il n'y a pas de définition consensuelle de sinusite récidivante. La seule retrouvée dans la littérature est dérivée de l'otite (trois en six mois ou quatre en un an)* »(4).

- « *Pour les pneumonies, il n'y a pas de définition internationalement admise ; deux épisodes en un an ou trois épisodes dans n'importe quel délai doivent être considérés comme entrant dans le cadre des pneumonies récidivantes à condition que la radio soit normale entre les épisodes* »(16).

- « *Pour les bronchiolites, trois épisodes dans les deux premières années de vie font parler d'asthme du nourrisson* »(17).

- « *Pour les laryngites, et les bronchites, il n'y a pas de définition internationalement admise* »(4).

Ces différentes définitions sont résumées dans le tableau 1(4).

Tableau 1: Définition du caractère récidivant des différentes infections respiratoires hautes et basses.

Otites :	Trois épisodes en six mois ou quatre épisodes en un an.
Angines :	Sept épisodes ou plus en un an ou dix épisodes dans les deux à trois dernières années.
Rhinopharyngites (après trois ans) :	Six épisodes fébriles.
Sinusites (après trois ans) :	Trois épisodes en six mois ou quatre en un an
Pneumonies :	Deux épisodes en un an ou trois épisodes dans n'importe quel délai (radio normale entre les épisodes).
Manifestations respiratoires basses obstructives (toux, gêne expiratoire et sibilant) chez un nourrisson :	Trois épisodes dans les deux premières années de vie font parler a priori d'asthme du nourrisson.

On remarque également que la plupart des études donnent des définitions par site infecté et s'intéressent peu au statut infectieux global de l'enfant en tant que tel.

Par ailleurs, de nombreuses études ont cherché à mettre en évidence les facteurs favorisant la répétition de ces infections :
Ils sont d'une part liés à l'individu :

- âge de début précoce des premiers épisodes(6),
- sexe masculin(6)(19)(20),
- carence martiale(6),
- allergie(6)(8)(21), antécédents familiaux d'allergie(8)(19)(20)(22), asthme(7)
- existence d'un reflux gastro-oesophagien(6),
- hypertrophie des végétations adénoïdes(6),
- présence d'une affection somatique grave(8),
- facteurs anatomiques (corps étranger, tumeur, adénopathies infectieuses ou tumorales, bronchectasie) (7)(21)

Et d'autre part liés à l'environnement :
- absence ou insuffisance d'allaitement maternel(6),
- manque d'ensoleillement(10),
- existence d'un tabagisme passif(6)(7)(8)(10)(21)(23)(24)(25),
- humidité, nettoyage de la maison au balai à poussières, insalubrité du domicile, pollution(7)(8)(10)
- phénomènes de résistance aux antibiotiques(7)(8),
- vie précoce en collectivité(6)(21),
- statut socio démographique des parents(8)(24), et statut socio-économique (25), précaires.
- altération de l'interaction entre une mère et son enfant qui conditionne la santé physique ultérieure de l'enfant(26).

Un des facteurs de risque d'infections répétées le plus étudié reste la crèche et donc l'entrée en collectivité précoce. Depuis une vingtaine d'années, nombre d'études en France et à l'étranger permettent d'attester de ces faits(9)(10)(27)(28)(29)(30) (31)(32).

La fréquence des infections est plus élevée chez les enfants d'âge préscolaire gardés en collectivité que chez les enfants élevés à domicile(8). En effet, la vie des jeunes enfants en collectivité s'accompagne d'un accroissement du risque infectieux, en particulier ORL et broncho-pulmonaire. Cela est lié au fait que *« les enfants ont une immunité moins développée, qu'ils sont porteurs bien plus souvent que les adultes de bactéries potentiellement pathogènes, et qu'ils peuvent s'infecter facilement les uns et les autres dans un milieu collectif, lequel exige des mesures accrues d'hygiène, surtout chez les enfants qui ont à être fréquemment changés »*(12). Strangert (1976)(33) montre que, sur une période de huit mois, les nourrissons en crèche collective présentent en moyenne cinq infections rebelles fébriles contre trois chez ceux qui sont gardés au domicile(12).

Cette incidence plus forte serait toutefois moins liée au mode de garde qu'au nombre d'enfants gardés. En effet, deux études américaines(34)(29) suggèrent que la présence de frères et sœurs à domicile peut avoir le même impact sur la fréquence des infections respiratoires que la garde en crèche.

L'excès de risque infectieux diminue avec l'âge et la durée de fréquentation de la crèche, témoignant d'une augmentation des défenses immunitaires des enfants, facilitée par la vie en collectivité. Une seule étude(35) s'intéresse à l'incidence des infections à l'âge scolaire en fonction du mode de garde des enfants avant leur scolarisation et montre que les enfants qui n'ont pas fréquenté de crèche sont plus souvent malades à un âge scolaire que les enfants mis en collectivité à un âge précoce.

De cette analyse précise de l'impact de l'entrée en crèche sur les infections dites à répétition, découle une donnée importante : *« il a été parfaitement démontré que les taux annuels de survenue d'infections respiratoires, d'otites moyennes aiguës et de consommation d'antibiotiques étaient parallèles et plus élevés au sein du groupe des enfants gardés en crèche* »(11). Ainsi les enfants gardés en crèche reçoivent plus souvent des antibiotiques que ceux gardés à domicile(12). Or, on touche là à une menace de santé publique majeure, comme nous le rappelle le plan national 2011-2016 d'alerte sur les antibiotiques(36), en raison du nombre croissant de situations d'impasse thérapeutique contre les infections bactériennes, du fait du développement des résistances aux antibiotiques. Il est également intéressant de souligner que parmi les pays européens, la France était, au début des années 2000, celui qui consommait le plus d'antibiotiques : avec environ 100 millions de prescriptions par an, dont 80% en ville(36). Or les principales situations cliniques responsables de l'augmentation de la prescription extra-hospitalière et de la consommation des antibiotiques sont les infections respiratoires hautes et basses, d'origine virale ou bactérienne(37).

Le plan d'alerte « *mise sur une stratégie de juste utilisation des antibiotiques et vise une réduction de la consommation d'antibiotiques de 25% en 5 ans. Pour ceci elle espère améliorer les règles de prise en charge par les antibiotiques; informer et former les professionnels de santé ; et sensibiliser la population aux enjeux d'une bonne prise en charge* »(36).

Afin de guider les praticiens dans la prescription des antibiotiques et limiter leur utilisation à tort, la Haute Autorité de Santé (HAS), la Caisse Nationale d'Assurance Maladie des Travailleurs Salariés (CNAMTS), la Caisse Nationale d'Assurance Maladie (CNAM), la Société Française de Pédiatrie (SFP), et la Société de Pathologie Infectieuse de Langue Française (SPILF) ont établi des recommandations et des guides pratiques pour la prise en charge des principales infections de l'enfant :

- Infections respiratoires hautes de l'enfant(38)
- Rhinopharyngite(39)
- Bronchiolite du nourrisson(40)
- Bronchite aigue(41)
- Otite moyenne aigue(42)
- Sinusite aigue(43)

Mais aussi un livret de sensibilisation pour les professionnels en charge de l'accueil des jeunes enfants, concernant les infections ORL et bronchiques(44), et un guide actualisé sur les résistances aux antibiotiques(45).

Face à un enfant qui présente des infections respiratoires anormalement fréquentes, un passage en revue des différentes étiologies vues précédemment doit être envisagé, avant de s'interroger sur un éventuel déficit immunitaire. En effet, même si la plupart des infections répétées sont d'origine virale, il ne faudrait pas oublier que chez certains enfants, elles peuvent être l'expression d'une pathologie sous-jacente ou d'un contexte défavorable.

Plusieurs études sont rassurantes quant à l'attitude à avoir face à des infections répétées(4)(21). Lorsque ces infections sont bénignes, il est assez rare qu'elles soient le reflet d'un déficit immunitaire avéré, ainsi il est exceptionnel que des otites moyennes aigues répétées isolées conduisent à découvrir un déficit immunitaire classique (13)(21). Dans l'immense majorité des cas, les examens complémentaires sont inutiles. L'essentiel est de rassurer, car cette pathologie se raréfie avec l'âge(6). « *La prise en charge de ces enfants ne doit jamais occulter le fait que l'histoire naturelle se fait vers la guérison, dans l'immense majorité des cas* »(4). Ainsi Alho et al.(46), en Finlande, ont rapporté le suivi pendant deux ans d'une cohorte de 222 enfants répondant aux définitions internationalement admises d'otites récidivantes qui n'avaient reçu aucun traitement spécifique ; seulement 4% ont développé une otite chronique et 12 % ont continué à présenter des otites moyennes aiguës récidivantes. De même, pour les infections respiratoires basses, on sait, aujourd'hui, que la grande majorité des nourrissons présentant des épisodes bronchiques sibilants répétés sont associés à des virus et n'évoluent pas vers la maladie asthmatique.

Il est exceptionnel qu'un déficit immunitaire se révèle uniquement par des infections respiratoires récidivantes, sans association à d'autres infections de localisations différentes.

Siegrist(21) dans son étude parue en 2001, précise les infections récidivantes qui doivent amener à dépister un déficit immunitaire : les otites à répétitions uniquement si elles sont associées à des infections broncho-pulmonaires, ou si elles deviennent chroniques ou persistent après l'âge de cinq ans ; les infections respiratoires (rhinopharyngite, laryngite, trachéite, bronchiolite, bronchite) d'origine présumée virale que si elles surviennent avant l'âge de trois mois, ou si leur évolution est particulièrement sévère. « *En dehors de ces conditions, il est plus utile de rechercher d'autres facteurs prédisposant comme l'atopie, l'hyperréactivité bronchique, l'exposition au tabagisme, la fréquentation de nombreux jeunes enfants (crèche) ou encore des facteurs anatomiques* »(21).
En revanche, l'infection pulmonaire mérite qu'on y prête une attention particulière car plus suspecte d'un déficit sous-jacent. « *Ainsi, une pneumonie avant l'âge de trois mois, ou un deuxième épisode de pneumonie, quel que soit l'âge, sont des indications absolues pour rechercher un déficit immunitaire* »(21). A noter, les complications d'infections ORL telles que la mastoïdite, l'abcès, la méningite bactérienne sont toujours suspectes. Ainsi

d'après Siegrist *« L'association « otites – sinusites– bronchopneumonies récidivantes » est particulièrement évocatrice d'un déficit immunitaire»*(21).

Ainsi le défi essentiel face à ces situations est d'identifier les enfants dont les infections récidivantes peuvent être le témoin d'une maladie sous-jacente, sans multiplier bilans et traitements inutiles chez ceux dont le développement immunitaire se déroule normalement.

Si un bilan est envisagé, Cohen et al.(4) donne des pistes de dépistage selon le site des infections répétées : quel que soit le site, une numération formule sanguine (NFS) à la recherche d'une lymphopénie ou neutropénie et dépister une carence en fer grâce au taux d'hémoglobine et au volume globulaire moyen (VGM).

- Un bilan allergologique : avant trois ans : IgE totales, IgE spécifiques soit ciblées, soit regroupées en kits (Trophatop®, Phadiatop® par exemple) ; et après trois ans : tests cutanés (prick test) ou recherche d'IgE spécifiques (Phadiatop®).

Puis selon le contexte :
- fibroscopie nasopharyngée : pour apprécier l'état des végétations et rechercher des signes indirects de reflux gastro-oesophagien (RGO);
- pHmétrie : à la recherche d'un RGO ;

Enfin selon le site :
- Pour les otites récidivantes : bilan initial avec NFS et un bilan allergologique. Puis secondairement, fibroscopie nasopharyngée. Et enfin troisièmement, pHmétrie et bilan immunitaire.

- Pour les rhinopharyngites récidivantes : même type de bilan complété précocement par une radio de thorax.
- Pour les angines récidivantes : aucun bilan n'est utile. « *En effet, il est exceptionnel que cette situation amène à découvrir une cause sous-jacente.* »(4)
- Pour les rhino-sinusites récidivantes : le bilan initial avec NFS, bilan allergologique, radio de thorax et test de la sueur. Secondairement, bilan immunologique, pHmétrie, et scanner à la recherche d'une malformation osseuse ou d'une polypose a minima. Puis troisièmement brossage ou biopsie de la muqueuse nasale afin d'éliminer une dyskinésie ciliaire primitive.
- Pour les infections respiratoires basses récidivantes, la recherche de la cause apparaît souvent comme fondamentale car la plus suspecte d'un déficit sous-jacent : pour cela, il est préférable d'adresser le patient pour un bilan spécialisé.

Au regard de toutes ces informations concernant les infections dites à répétition chez l'enfant, il est intéressant de se questionner sur leur impact en médecine générale: quelle est la proportion d'enfants faisant des infections plus fréquemment que les autres en pratique de ville et comment évoluent les dites infections sur 10 ans ?

Avec quelle fréquence les différents sites infectieux sont-ils atteints et quelles combinaisons de sites infectieux sont retrouvées chez les enfants souvent infectés ?

Quelles comorbidités peuvent influencer ces infections fréquentes ?

II. OBJECTIFS :

L'objectif principal de cette étude est de décrire le statut infectieux de 1014 enfants suivis pendant 10 ans grâce à la réalisation d'une typologie.

Les objectifs secondaires sont de rechercher des critères permettant de repérer les enfants faisant des infections répétées de manière inhabituelle, et de poser les bases de leur repérage. Et d'analyser la prescription d'antibiotiques par classes de la typologie

III. MATERIEL ET MÉTHODE :

A. TYPE D'ÉTUDE :

Étude descriptive rétrospective
Analyse en composante principale et classification ascendante hiérarchique

B. ANALYSE BIBLIOGRAPHIQUE :

Les moteurs de recherche bibliographiques utilisés :
- Pub Med
- Refdoc
- Sudoc
- Google Scholar
- Google

Les sites consultés :
- La revue du praticien
- Médecine et enfance
- Haute Autorité de Santé (HAS)
- Caisse Nationale d'Assurance Maladie des Travailleurs Salariés (CNAMTS)
- Caisse Nationale d'Assurance Maladie (CNAM)
- Société Française de Pédiatrie (SFP)
- Société de Pathologie Infectieuse de Langue Française (SPILF)

Les mots clés utilisés en français :
- Médecine générale

- Pédiatrie
- Enfants, nourrissons
- Infections à répétition
- Infections récidivantes
- Infections récurrentes
- Infections répétées
- Crèche, collectivité, mode de garde
- Déficit immunitaire

Les mots clés utilisés en anglais :
- Général practice
- Pediatrics
- Infant, child
- Recurrent infections
- Repeated infections
- Nursery, child care, custody mode
- Immunologic deficiency syndromes

Résultats et sélection des articles :

Sur les 108 éléments bibliographiques retrouvés avec les mots clefs ci-dessus, seuls 49 ont été retenus pour la bibliographie, centrés sur les infections dites à répétition chez les enfants sains.

C. MATERIEL :

1. Observatoire de Médecine Générale (OMG) :

La Société Française de Médecine Générale (SFMG) a créé en 1993 un réseau de médecins répartis sur toute la France, utilisant un dossier médical informatisé structuré, ayant abouti à la création de l'Observatoire de Médecine Générale (OMG)(47). Celui-ci résulte du travail des médecins investigateurs qui fournissent les données, et le Département d'Information Médical de la SFMG qui les traitent. Le recueil des données se fait par les médecins investigateurs, en temps réel pendant leur consultation, à l'aide d'un outil spécifique intégré dans le logiciel du médecin : le Dictionnaire des Résultats de Consultation (DRC). Lors de chaque consultation, le médecin recueille les diagnostics des problèmes pris en charge lors de la consultation (cf. annexe 1).

a) Base de données Diogène :

Diogène est une base de données médicale qui comprend les caractéristiques :
- des médecins : genre, âge, lieu et mode d'exercice, secteur conventionnel.
- des patients : genre, âge, mode de vie, antécédents médicaux.
- des consultations : diagnostics, code suivi (nouveau diagnostic, diagnostic persistant), prescriptions des examens para cliniques et médicaments.

En 2011, la base recense plus de 870 000 patients pris en charge lors de 8 millions de séances, avec 10 millions de résultats de consultations et 20 millions de prescriptions médicamenteuses.

b) Éléments absents de la base :

Certains éléments ne sont pas décrits dans la base de données :
- la catégorie socio-professionnelle de l'enfant et/ou de sa famille
- le mode de garde entre zéro et trois ans : crèche, crèche familiale ou domicile

2. Base d'étude et variables utilisées :

Sélection de dix pathologies infectieuses fréquentes en médecine générale (cf. annexe n°2) et recueil du nombre de consultations pour ces différentes pathologies, par enfants, par an, sur 10 ans.

Choix des variables indépendantes:
En dehors du genre et du lieu de vie, nous avons étudié les autres variables en fonction de trois groupes d'âges : 0-2 (préscolaire) / 3-5 (maternelle) / 6-10 (primaire).

Tableau 2: Variables choisies.

Variables	Modalités
Genre :	Garçon / Fille
Age, date de naissance :	1999, 2000, 2001
Lieu de vie :	Urbain / semi-rural / rural
Comorbidités : - Asthme - Eczéma - Rhinite - Dermatose - Reflux gastro- oesophagien - Anémie ferriprive –carence martiale	Oui / Non Pour chaque comorbidité par classe d'âge
Nombre de résultats de consultation infectieux :	Nombre de RC différents par classe d'âge (modalités à définir)
RC infectieux : (cf. annexe n° 3) ⇨ ANGINE (AMYGDALITE - PHARYNGITE) ⇨ BRONCHITE AIGUË ⇨ DIARRHEE NAUSEE VOMISSEMENT ⇨ ÉTAT AFÉBRILE ⇨ ÉTAT FÉBRILE ⇨ OTITE MOYENNE ⇨ PNEUMOPATHIE AIGUE ⇨ RHINOPHARYNGITE –RHUME ⇨ SINUSITE ⇨ TOUX	Nombre de RC différents pour chaque RC infectieux sélectionnés et par classe d'âge (modalités à définir)
Code suivi :	Rapport du nombre de cas nouveaux sur le nombre de cas persistants par classe d'âge (modalités à définir)
Nombre d'antibiotiques :	Nombre de fois où il y a prescription d'antibiotiques par classe d'âge (modalité à définir)
Nombre de séances :	Nombre total de séances par an réparties par classe d'âge (modalités à définir)

D. METHODE:

Dans un premier temps, nous avons réalisé une analyse descriptive d'une population de 1014 enfants nés entre 1999 et 2001 et suivis pendant 10 ans par 53 médecins de l'observatoire de médecine générale (OMG) : description de leurs pathologies infectieuses, prescription ou non d'un traitement antibiotique, nombre d'actes réalisés par an et repérage des comorbidités sélectionnées.

Ceci permettant de déterminer les modalités des variables qui serviront à l'analyse factorielle.

Dans un second temps, nous avons réalisé une analyse en composante principale et classification ascendante hiérarchique.

Variables actives : nombre de résultats de consultation infectieux par classe d'âge, nombre de comorbidités globales.

Variables illustratives : commune, genre, médecin traitant, détail de chaque comorbidité, le nombre de résultats de consultation infectieux différents, détail de chaque pathologie infectieuse.

Nous avons créé la variable « Médecin Traitant » en considérant que le médecin généraliste était le médecin traitant s'il avait vu l'enfant au moins 4 fois pour « examen systématique » entre 0 et 2 ans, (soit au moins 3 fois entre 0 et 11 mois et au moins une fois entre 12 et 35 mois.)

Enfin pour répondre en partie à l'objectif secondaire, nous avons réalisé une courbe ROC pour choisir la meilleure classe de la typologie permettant le repérage des enfants infectés de manière inhabituelle.

Méthode d'analyse des données envisagée :

Analyse descriptive et factorielle réalisée avec le logiciel de statistique SPAD version 7.4

Analyse descriptive par tableaux croisés dynamiques, sous Excel.

Construction des courbes de ROC sous SAS 9.2

Nous avons utilisés les médianes et quartiles, moyennes et écart-types.

Le test non paramétrique de Wilcoxon, et le test exact de Fischer.

IV. ANALYSE DESCRIPTIVE :

A. LES PATIENTS :

Notre échantillon issu de la base de données de l'OMG, contient 1014 patients nés entre 1999 et 2001, avec une répartition équivalente entre les filles et les garçons (p=0,39).

Tableau 3: Nombre de naissances selon l'année et le sexe.

Années de naissance	F	G	TOTAL	Années de naissance	F	G	TOTAL
1999	156	215	371	1999	34,4%	38,3%	36,6%
2000	165	185	350	2000	36,4%	33,0%	34,5%
2001	132	161	293	2001	29,1%	28,7%	28,9%
Total	453	561	1014	Total	100,0%	100,0%	100,0%

B. LES ACTES :

Ces patients ont généré 14 956 actes dans la classe d'âge 0-2 ans, 10 122 dans la classe d'âge 3-5 ans et 10 693 actes dans la classe d'âge 6-10 ans, soit au total 35 771 actes tout âge confondu et quelle que soit la nature de l'acte.

La médiane des actes par classe d'âge est de 12 entre 0 et 2 ans (soit un acte en moyenne tous les 2 mois) alors qu'elle n'est que de 9 entre 3 et 5 ans et entre 6 et 10 ans (soit un acte en moyenne tous les 4 mois entre 3 et 5 ans et un acte tous les 6 mois et demi entre 6 et 10 ans).

Tableau 4: Nombre d'actes médians par classe d'âge.

Age	0-2 ans	3-5 ans	6-10 ans
1er quartile inclus	4	4	5
Médiane	12	9	9
3ème quartile inclus	23	14	14

Le test de Wilcoxon ne montre pas de différence statistiquement significative entre les garçons et les filles quelle que soit la classe d'âge (p=0,5).

C. LES RESULTATS DE CONSULTATION :

Dans 90% des cas, il n'y a qu'un seul résultat de consultation (RC) par acte.

Le nombre de résultats de consultation différents utilisés est de 51, représentant 90% des 221 RC utilisés[2]. Les dix résultats de consultation infectieux sélectionnés représentent en fréquence d'utilisation, 81 % de tous les résultats de consultation utilisés (cf. annexe n°2).

Le RC « examen systématique » représente 14% des RC utilisés et 11% des RC entre 0 et 2 ans, 5,65% entre 3 et 5 ans et 17,50% entre 6 et 10 ans. (Fig.1).

---

[2] Le Dictionnaire des Résultats de Consultation contient 277 définitions

Figure 1: Répartition des différents types de résultats de consultation selon la classe d'âge.

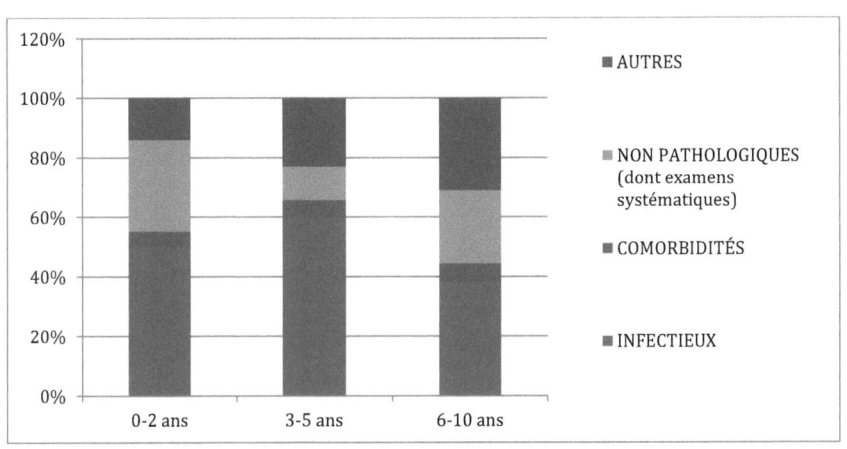

D. LES RESULTAT DE CONSULTATION INFECTIEUX :

1. En fonction du sexe :

Tableau 5: Répartition de la population en fonction du sexe.

	Effectif		Moyenne		Écart type (N-1)		1er quartile		Médiane		3ème quartile	
Sexe:	F	G	F	G	F	G	F	G	F	G	F	G
0-2 ans	453	561	8	8,05	8	7,56	2	2	6	6	12	12
3-5 ans	453	561	6,34	6,08	5,43	5,11	2	2	5	5	9	9
6-10 ans	453	561	4,78	4,20	4,33	4	1	1	4	3	7	6

Le tableau 5 montre une dispersion autour de la moyenne importante et une décroissance progressive des médianes des RC infectieux en fonction de l'âge.

Le test de Wilcoxon n'a pas montré de différence statistiquement significative ente les garçons et les filles, pour la classe d'âge 0-2 ans (p=0,929) ni pour la classe d'âge 3-5 ans (p=0,572). En revanche il existe une différence statistiquement significative concernant la classe d'âge 6-10 ans (p=0,023), en faveur des filles.

2. En fonction du lieu d'habitation:

Tableau 6: Répartition de la population selon leur lieu d'habitation.

Modalités	Effectifs	Pourcentages
Rural	184	18%
Semi-Rural	257	25%
Urbain	573	57%
Ensemble	1014	100%

Plus de la moitié des enfants de l'échantillon sont issus d'un milieu urbain.

Tableaux 7: Comparaison de la distribution de la population en milieu rural et urbain en fonction de l'âge (en valeur absolue et en pourcentage)

	0-2 ans		3-5 ans		6-10 ans	
	RURAL	URBAIN	RURAL	URBAIN	RURAL	URBAIN
1er quartile	38	185	38	191	44	193
2e quartile	34	162	54	150	60	144
3e quartile	55	119	45	128	45	134
4e quartile	57	107	47	104	35	102
Total	184	573	184	573	184	573

	0-2 ans		3-5 ans		6-10 ans	
	RURAL	URBAIN	RURAL	URBAIN	RURAL	URBAIN
1er quartile	21%	32%	21%	33%	24%	34%
2e quartile	18%	28%	29%	26%	33%	25%
3e quartile	30%	21%	24%	22%	24%	23%
4e quartile	31%	19%	26%	18%	19%	18%
Total	100%	100%	100%	100%	100%	100%

Concernant le nombre d'infections, le test de Wilcoxon a montré une différence statistiquement significative en faveur des enfants issus d'un milieu urbain par rapport à ceux issus d'un milieu rural pour les classes d'âge 0-2 ans ($p=8 \times 10^{-6}$) et 3-5 ans (p=0,005). En revanche, il n'existe pas de différence statistiquement significative entre 6 et 10 ans (p=0,058).

3. En fonction de la classe d'âge :

Tableau 8: Résultats de consultation infectieux par classe d'âge.

RC infectieux	0-2 ans	3-5 ans	6-10 ans	RC infectieux	% 0-2	% 3-5	% 6-10
ÉTAT FÉBRILE	2160	1609	1377	ÉTAT FÉBRILE	26%	25%	30%
RHINOPHARYNGITE - RHUME	2135	1321	861	RHINOPHARYNGITE - RHUME	26%	21%	19%
ÉTAT MORBIDE AFÉBRILE	1197	940	765	ÉTAT MORBIDE AFÉBRILE	15%	15%	17%
OTITE MOYENNE	1060	767	389	OTITE MOYENNE	13%	12%	8%
BRONCHITE AIGUË	540	327	164	BRONCHITE AIGUË	7%	5%	4%
ANGINE (AMYGDALITE - PHARYNGITE)	522	740	507	ANGINE (AMYGDALITE - PHARYNGITE)	6%	12%	11%
TOUX	344	377	224	TOUX	4%	6%	5%
DIARRHÉE NAUSÉE VOMISSEMENTS	249	224	266	DIARRHÉE NAUSÉE VOMISSEMENTS	3%	4%	6%
PNEUMOPATHIE AIGUË	17	26	15	PNEUMOPATHIE AIGUË	0%	0%	0%
SINUSITE	3	15	18	SINUSITE	0%	0%	0%
TOTAL	8227	6346	4586	TOTAL	100%	100%	100%

Quel que soit l'âge, les trois pathologies infectieuses les plus retrouvées sont l'état fébrile, la rhinopharyngite et l'état afébrile. Ces trois RC infectieux représentent à peu près les 2/3 des RC infectieux utilisés (respectivement 67% entre 0 et 2 ans, 61% entre 3 et 5 ans et 65% entre 6 et 10 ans).

Les RC « pneumopathie » et « sinusite » sont exceptionnels quel que soit l'âge.

Tableau 9: Répartition des moyennes des résultats de consultation infectieux entre 0 et 2 ans.

0-2 ans		
Pathologies infectieuses	Moyenne	Écart type
État fébrile	2,102	2,376
Rhinopharyngite	2,077	2,482
État afébrile	1,172	1,911
Otite	1,028	1,875
Bronchite	0,533	1,148
Angine	0,511	1,050
Toux	0,336	0,715
Diarrhée Vomissements	0,244	0,582
Pneumopathie	0,017	0,136
Sinusite	0,003	0,054

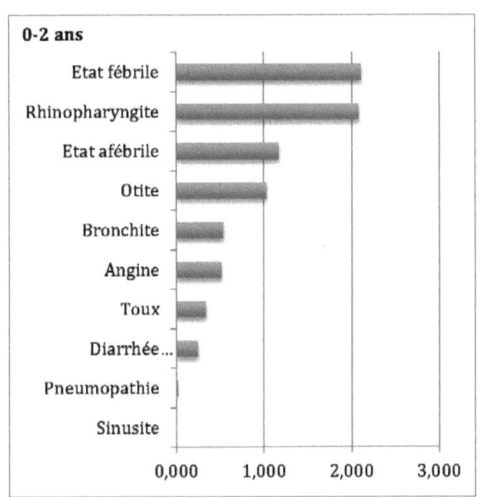

Chaque enfant âgé de 0 à 2 ans fait en moyenne sur cette période de deux ans, deux états fébriles, deux rhinopharyngites, un état afébrile, et une otite. Un enfant sur deux fait une bronchite et/ou une angine. Un enfant sur trois présente un épisode de toux et un enfant sur quatre présente un épisode de diarrhée vomissements. Les diagnostics de pneumopathie et de sinusite concernent moins d'un enfant sur 100).

Tableau 10: Répartition des moyennes des résultats de consultation infectieux entre 3 et 5 ans.

3-5 ans		
Pathologies infectieuses	Moyenne	Ecart type
Etat fébrile	1,566	1,751
Rhinopharyngite	1,289	1,835
Etat afébrile	0,917	1,575
Otite	0,751	1,240
Angine	0,724	1,259
Toux	0,371	0,849
Bronchite	0,321	0,768
Diarrhée Vomissements	0,218	0,504
Pneumopathie	0,026	0,158
Sinusite	0,015	0,136

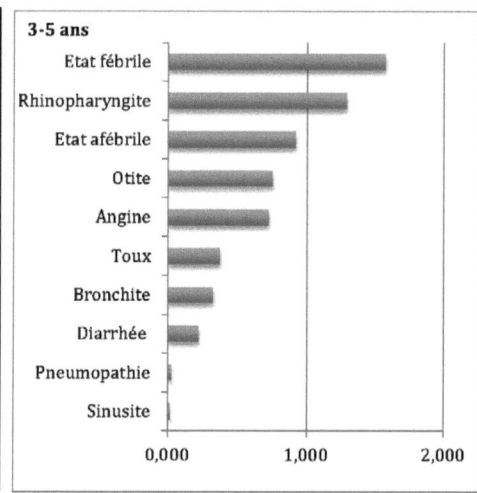

Chaque enfant âgé de 3 à 5 ans fait en moyenne sur cette période de deux ans, un à deux épisodes d'états fébriles, une rhinopharyngite, et un état afébrile. Deux enfants sur trois présentent une otite et/ou une angine. Un enfant sur trois présente un épisode de toux et/ou une bronchite, et une enfant sur cinq présente un épisode de diarrhée vomissements. Les diagnostics de pneumopathie et de sinusite restent très rares, respectivement un enfant sur cinquante et un enfant sur cent.

Tableau 11 : Répartition des moyennes des résultats de consultation infectieux entre 6 et 10 ans.

6-10 ans		
Pathologies infectieuses	Moyenne	Ecart type
Etat fébrile	1,336	1,587
Rhinopharyngite	0,836	1,367
Etat afébrile	0,742	1,356
Angine	0,496	0,978
Otite	0,378	0,807
Diarrhée Vomissements	0,260	0,565
Toux	0,221	0,575
Bronchite	0,159	0,549
Sinusite	0,017	0,136
Pneumopathie	0,015	0,121

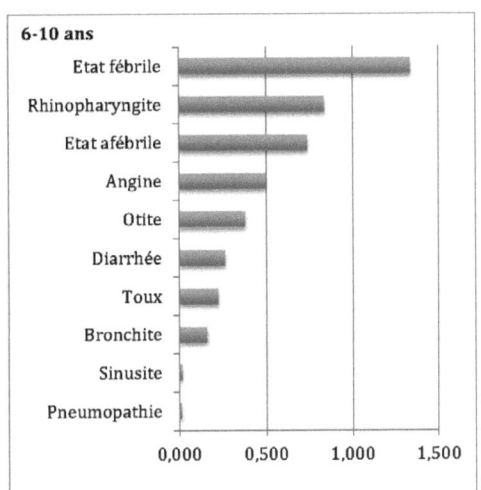

Chaque enfant âgé de 6 à 10 ans fait en moyenne sur cette période de quatre ans, un à deux états fébriles. Quatre enfants sur cinq présentent une rhinopharyngite et/ou un état afébrile. Un enfant sur deux fait une angine. Un enfant sur quatre fait une otite. Un enfant sur trois présente un épisode de diarrhée vomissements. Un enfant sur huit présente une bronchite. Un enfant sur cent fait une sinusite et/ou une pneumopathie.

Ainsi la distribution des RC infectieux par classe d'âge est assez similaire mais les écarts sont moins importants avec l'âge.

4. En fonction des trois résultats de consultation représentant les deux tiers des pathologies infectieuses :

a) État fébrile (EF) :

<u>Tableau 12 :</u> Distribution de la fréquence de l'état fébrile par classe d'âge.

Nombre de patients	0-2 ans	3-5 ans	6-10 ans
1 EF	0	252	264
2 EF	136	168	168
3 EF	124	103	95
4 EF	73	68	41
5 EF	52	34	30
6 EF	36	22	11
7 EF	18	6	5
8 EF	15	3	3
9 EF	11	2	2
10 EF	4	1	0
11 EF	4	1	0
12 EF	2	1	0
13 EF	0	0	1
Total	475	661	620

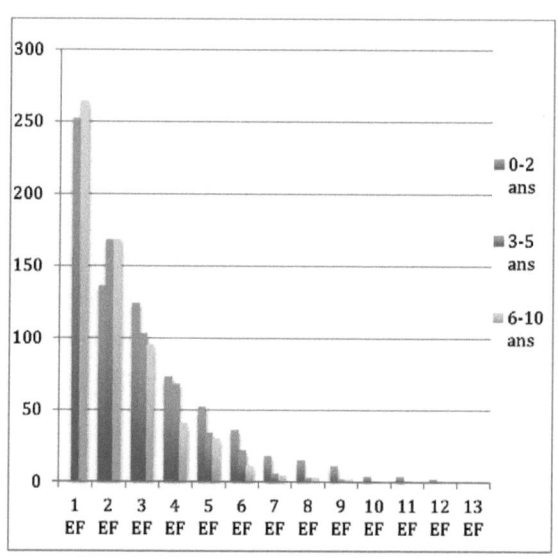

Sur les 1014 enfants, 46,8% des enfants font un ou plusieurs états fébriles entre 0 et 2 ans, 65,2% entre 3 et 5 ans et 61,2% entre 6 et 10 ans. Parmi ces enfants qui font des états fébriles, un peu plus de la moitié des 0-2 ans (55%) vont faire deux ou trois états fébriles sur la période, les 2/3 des 3-5 ans, et 70% des 6-10 ans vont faire 1 ou 2 états fébriles sur la période.

b) **Rhinopharyngite (RPH):**

<u>Tableau 13:</u> Distribution de la fréquence de la rhinopharyngite par classe d'âge.

Nombre de patients	0-2 ans	3-5 ans	6-10 ans
1 RPH	0	246	215
2 RPH	146	118	96
3 RPH	100	63	55
4 RPH	72	52	28
5 RPH	54	28	15
6 RPH	38	13	4
7 RPH	12	8	3
8 RPH	30	7	3
9 RPH	0	5	1
10 RPH	4	3	0
11 RPH	3	1	1
12 RPH	0	1	0
13 RPH	4	0	0
14 RPH	1	0	0
15 RPH	3	0	0
Total	467	545	421

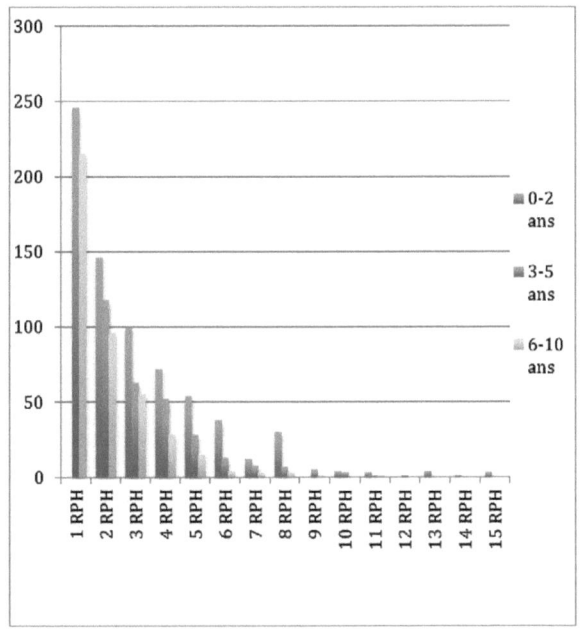

Sur les 1014 enfants, 46% des enfants font une ou plusieurs rhinopharyngites entre 0 et 2 ans, 53,7% entre 3 et 5 ans et 41,5% entre 6 et 10 ans. Parmi ces enfants qui font des rhinopharyngites, la moitié des enfants âgés de 0 à 2 ans vont faire 2 à 3 rhinopharyngites sur la période, près de la moitié des 3-5 ans (45%) et des 6-10 ans (51%) ne feront qu'une seule rhinopharyngite sur la période et 80% des 3-5 ans et 90% des 6-10 ans, pas plus de 3 sur la période.

c) **État afébrile (EA) :**

Tableau 14: Distribution de la fréquence de l'état afébrile par classe d'âge.

Nombre de patients	0-2 ans	3-5 ans	6-10 ans
1 EA	0	212	225
2 EA	95	90	89
3 EA	78	51	32
4 EA	24	31	17
5 EA	22	17	14
6 EA	16	9	6
7 EA	10	3	2
8 EA	11	4	2
9 EA	0	4	3
10 EA	2	0	1
11 EA	2	3	0
12 EA	1	0	1
13 EA	0	0	0
14 EA	1	0	0
15 EA	0	0	0
16 EA	1	0	0
Total	263	424	392

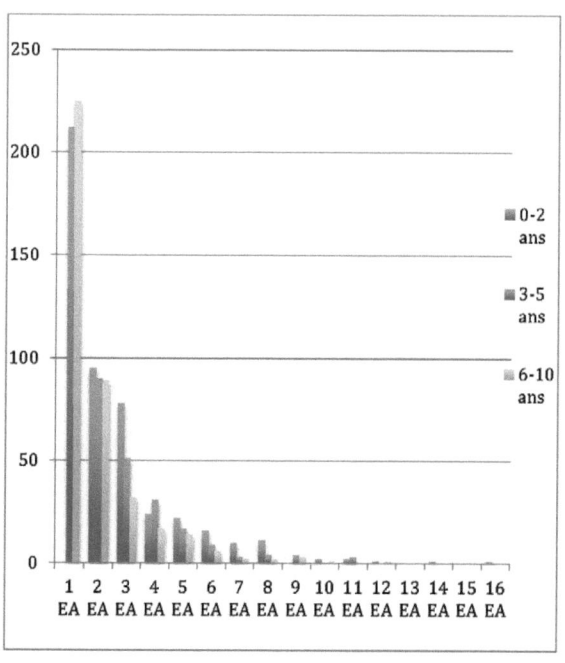

Sur les 1014 enfants, 25,9% enfants font un ou plusieurs états afébriles entre 0 et 2 ans, 41,8% entre 3 et 5 ans et 38,6% entre 6 et 10 ans. Parmi les enfants qui font des états afébriles, les ¾ des enfants âgés de 0 à 2 ans font 2 à 4 états afébriles sur la période, la moitié des 3-5 ans et un peu plus que la moitié (57%) des 6-10 ans n'en feront qu'un sur la période.

Au total, les trois pathologies les plus fréquentes, représentées par l'état fébrile, la rhinopharyngite et l'état afébrile, ont une distribution similaire en fonction des trois classes d'âge. Leur fréquence est très élevée chez les 0-2 ans, avec une distribution assez étalée, tandis que pour les 3-10 ans, la fréquence diminue plus rapidement.

5. En fonction du caractère aigüe ou persistant des résultats de consultation infectieux :

Pour chaque RC il est possible de préciser s'il s'agit d'un nouvel évènement (N) ou d'un évènement persistant (P). Quand le rapport N/P est supérieur à 1, alors les pathologies sont aiguës, et quand le rapport est proche de 1, il s'agit de pathologies plus souvent revues par le praticien (taux de retouche).

Tableau 15 : Rapport N/P des différentes pathologies infectieuses étudiées.

Classe d'âge	Pathologies infectieuses	N	P	N/P
0-2 ans	ANGINE (AMYGDALITE - PHARYNGITE)	518	50	10,4
	BRONCHITE AIGUË	540	158	3,4
	DIARRHÉE NAUSÉE VOMISSEMENTS	247	37	6,7
	ÉTAT FÉBRILE	2131	380	5,6
	ÉTAT MORBIDE AFÉBRILE	1188	195	6,1
	OTITE MOYENNE	1042	276	3,8
	PNEUMOPATHIE AIGUË	17	10	1,7
	RHINOPHARYNGITE - RHUME	2106	423	5,0
	SINUSITE	3	2	1,5
	TOUX	341	100	3,4
3-5 ans	ANGINE (AMYGDALITE - PHARYNGITE)	734	49	15,0
	BRONCHITE AIGUË	326	59	5,5
	DIARRHÉE NAUSÉE VOMISSEMENTS	221	28	7,9
	ÉTAT FÉBRILE	1588	249	6,4
	ÉTAT MORBIDE AFÉBRILE	930	99	9,4
	OTITE MOYENNE	762	146	5,2
	PNEUMOPATHIE AIGUË	26	22	1,2
	RHINOPHARYNGITE - RHUME	1307	223	5,9
	SINUSITE	15	4	3,8
	TOUX	376	91	4,1
6-10 ans	ANGINE (AMYGDALITE - PHARYNGITE)	503	37	13,6
	BRONCHITE AIGUË	161	27	6,0
	DIARRHÉE NAUSÉE VOMISSEMENTS	264	14	18,9
	ÉTAT FÉBRILE	1355	131	10,3
	ÉTAT MORBIDE AFÉBRILE	752	48	15,7
	OTITE MOYENNE	383	59	6,5
	PNEUMOPATHIE AIGUË	15	9	1,7
	RHINOPHARYNGITE - RHUME	848	95	8,9
	SINUSITE	17	11	1,5
	TOUX	224	79	2,8

Le taux de retouche pour les pathologies les plus fréquentes est faible et s'accentue avec l'âge.

6. Répartition du nombre d'infections par quartile et par classes d'âge :

Tableau 16 : Répartition par quartiles (en valeur absolue et en pourcentage).

Quartiles	Classes d'âge					
	0- 2 ans		3-5 ans		6-10 ans	
1er quartile	0-2 RC	273	0-2 RC	284	0-1 RC	298
2ème quartile	3-6 RC	254	3-5 RC	249	2-4 RC	295
3ème quartile	7-11 RC	226	6-9 RC	255	5-7 RC	226
4ème quartile	12 et plus RC	261	10 et plus RC	226	8 et plus RC	195
Total		1014		1014		1014

Quartiles	Classes d'âge					
	0- 2 ans		3-5 ans		6-10 ans	
1er quartile	0-2 RC	27%	0-2 RC	28%	0-1 RC	29%
2ème quartile	3-6 RC	25%	3-5 RC	25%	2-4 RC	29%
3ème quartile	7-11 RC	22%	6-9 RC	25%	5-7 RC	22%
4ème quartile	12 et plus RC	26%	10 et plus RC	22%	8 et plus RC	19%
Total		100%		100%		100%

Le nombre de RC infectieux par quartile diminue avec l'âge.

7. Répartition des enfants en fonction du nombre d'infections totales :

Nous avons cherché à savoir comment évoluaient dans le temps les enfants qui faisaient beaucoup d'infections entre 0 et 2 ans (quartiles 3 et 4 de la population 0-2 ans).

Tableau 17: Évolution du 4ème quartile de la population 0-2 ans, à 3-5 ans et 6 10 ans.

Q4 0-2 ans	3-5 ans	6-10 ans
Q1 (0-2 RC)	5%	13%
Q2 (3-6 RC)	22%	34%
Q3 (7-11 RC)	30%	24%
Q4 (>11 RC)	44%	29%

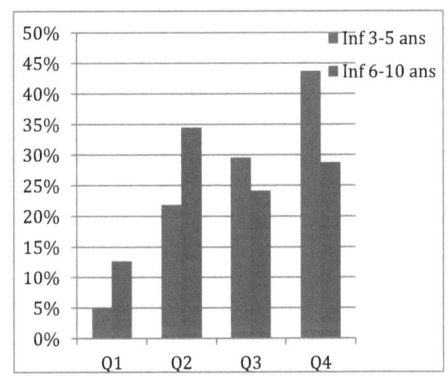

Tableau 18: Évolution du 3ème quartile de la population 0-2 ans, à 3-5 ans et 6-10 ans.

Q3 0-2 ans	3-5 ans	6-10 ans
Q1 (0-2 RC)	17%	30%
Q2 (3-6 RC)	23%	26%
Q3 (7-11 RC)	34%	23%
Q4 (>11 RC)	25%	22%

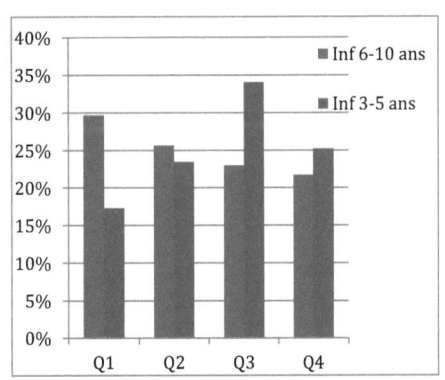

Les tableaux ci-dessus montrent que 29% des enfants appartenant au 4ème quartile entre 0 et 2 ans, appartiennent également au 4ème quartile entre 6 et 10

ans, tandis que 47% de ces enfants passent dans le 1er ou le 2ème quartile entre 6 et 10 ans.

De plus les enfants appartenant au 3ème quartile entre 0 et 2 ans se répartissent de façon quasi équivalente entre les quatre quartiles entre 6 et 10 ans.

8. Nombre de résultats de consultation infectieux différents par enfants :

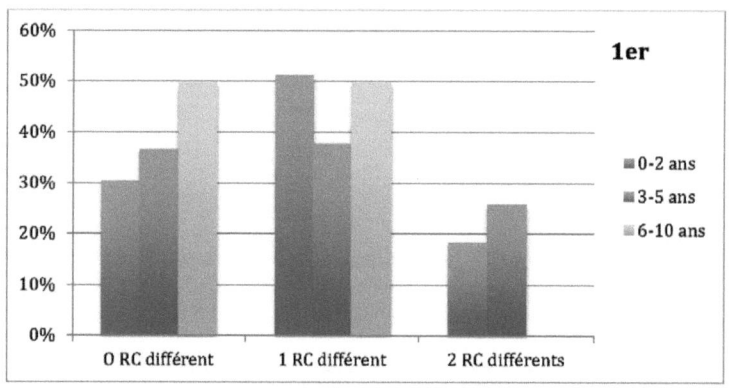

Figure 2 : Nombre de RC infectieux différents en fonction du 1er quartile du groupe 0-2 ans.

Figure 3 : Nombre de RC infectieux différents en fonction du 2ème quartile du groupe 0-2 ans.

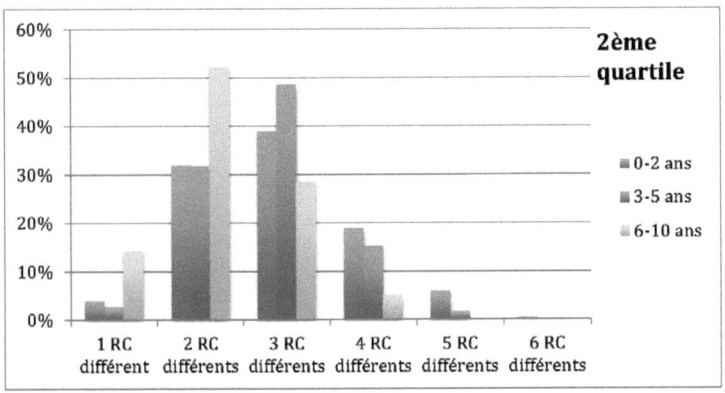

Figure 4: Nombre de RC infectieux différents en fonction du 3ème quartile du groupe 0-2 ans.

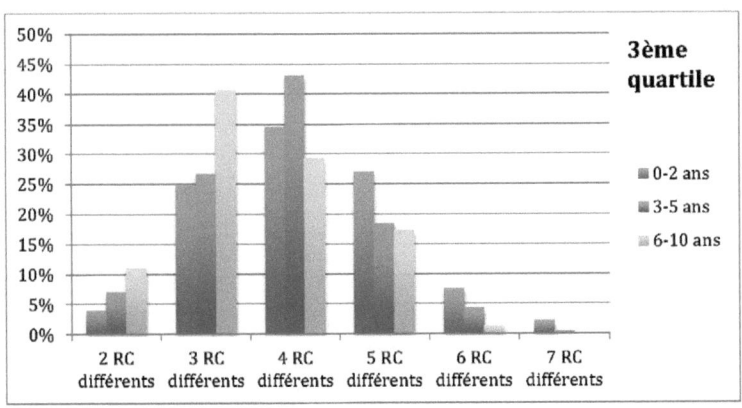

Figure 5 : Nombre de RC infectieux différents en fonction du 4ème quartile du groupe 0-2 ans.

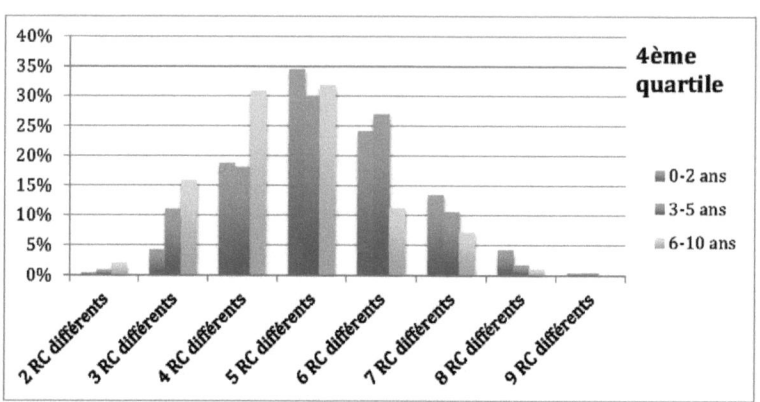

Quelle que soit la classe d'âge, plus les enfants font des infections (4ème quartile), plus le nombre de RC infectieux différents sur la période est élevé. Ce nombre de RC infectieux différents diminue en fonction du nombre d'infections, et se décale progressivement.

E. DISTRIBUTION DES COMORBIDITES :

Tableau 19 : Type de comorbidités par tranche d'âge (valeurs absolues et pourcentages).

Comorbidités	0-2 ans	3-5 ans	6-10 ans	Comorbidités	0-2 ans	3-5 ans	6-10 ans
Sans comorbidités	583	670	712	Sans comorbidités	57%	66%	70%
Dermatose	210	145	141	Dermatose	21%	14%	14%
Eczéma	168	96	108	Eczéma	17%	9%	11%
Asthme	90	97	100	Asthme	9%	10%	10%
Rhinite	92	92	108	Rhinite	9%	9%	11%
RGO	50	7	17	RGO	5%	1%	2%
Carence martiale	26	19	7	Carence martiale	3%	2%	1%

Les dermatoses diminuent de 30% et l'eczéma de moitié entre les 0-2 ans et les 3-10 ans. L'asthme et la rhinite restent stables tout au long des 10 ans. Le RGO et la carence martiale touchent moins de 5% des enfants de l'échantillon.

Tableau 20: Comorbidités selon la classe d'âge et le sexe (valeurs absolues et pourcentages).

Comorbidités	Classes d'âge	Garçons	Filles	Comorbidités	Classes d'âge	% Garçons	% Filles
Asthme	0-2 ans	66	24	Asthme	0-2 ans	11,8	5,3
	3-5 ans	64	33		3-5 ans	11,4	7,3
	6-10 ans	66	34		6-10 ans	11,8	7,51
Dermatose	0-2 ans	115	95	Dermatose	0-2 ans	20,5	21,0
	3-5 ans	79	66		3-5 ans	14,1	14,6
	6-10 ans	87	54		6-10 ans	15,5	11,9
Eczéma	0-2 ans	98	70	Eczéma	0-2 ans	17,5	15,5
	3-5 ans	56	40		3-5 ans	10,0	8,8
	6-10 ans	60	48		6-10 ans	10,7	10,6
Rhinite	0-2 ans	48	44	Rhinite	0-2 ans	8,6	9,7
	3-5 ans	59	33		3-5 ans	10,5	7,3
	6-10 ans	60	48		6-10 ans	10,7	10,6
RGO	0-2 ans	32	18	RGO	0-2 ans	5,7	4,0
	3-5 ans	5	2		3-5 ans	0,9	0,4
	6-10 ans	11	6		6-10 ans	2,0	1,3
Carence martiale	0-2 ans	23	3	Carence martiale	0-2 ans	4,1	0,7
	3-5 ans	11	8		3-5 ans	2,0	1,8
	6-10 ans	3	4		6-10 ans	0,5	0,9

La répartition entre les filles et les garçons est comparable concernant cinq des six comorbidités étudiées (dermatose, eczéma, rhinite, RGO et carence martiale). La seule différence statistiquement significative concerne l'asthme : les garçons sont plus atteints que les filles quel que soit l'âge (p=0,0003 entre 0 et 2 ans ; p=0,031 entre 3 et 5 ans et p=0,025 entre 6 et 10 ans).

F. MEDECIN TRAITANT :

1. Généralités

Rappel : nous avons considéré que le médecin généraliste était le médecin traitant s'il avait vu l'enfant au moins 4 fois pour « examen systématique » entre 0 et 2 ans, (soit au moins 3 fois entre 0 et 11 mois et au moins une fois entre 12 et 35 mois.)

Tableau 21: Répartition des enfants en fonction de leur médecin traitant

Médecin traitant	Total	Total (%)
OUI	522	51%
NON	492	49%
Total général	1014	100%

Parmi les 1014 patients de l'échantillon, 522 sont suivis par leur médecin traitant et 492 enfants par un autre médecin, soit une répartition à peu près équivalente.

Tableau 22: Test de Wilcoxon pour la recherche d'une différence entre le fait que l'enfant soit suivi ou non par son généraliste.

RC INF	MT: NON	MT: OUI	valeur de p
Moyenne observée 0-2 ans	4,848	11,011	0,000
Moyenne observée 3-5 ans	4,870	7,450	0,000
Moyenne observée 6-10 ans	4,077	4,820	0,001

Les tests de Wilcoxon ont montré qu'il existait une différence statistiquement significative concernant la prise en charge des RC infectieux en faveur du médecin traitant versus un autre médecin et ce quel que soit l'âge.

2. Lieu d'exercice :

Tableau 23: Médecin traitant en fonction du lieu d'exercice

Modalités	MT=NON	MT=OUI	Total
Rural	77	107	184
Semi-R	80	177	257
Urbain	335	238	573
Ensemble	492	522	1014

Modalités	MT=NON	MT=OUI	Total
Rural	42%	58%	100%
Semi-R	31%	69%	100%
Urbain	58%	42%	100%
Ensemble	49%	51%	100%

En région rurale et semi-rurale les enfants sont majoritairement suivis par leur médecin traitant (plus de 55%). Cette position est inverse en milieu urbain (42%).

G. SYNTHESE :

Tableau 24: Tableau de synthèse.

Variables	Valeur absolue			Pourcentage			Moyenne			Médiane		
	0-2 ans	3-5 ans	6-10 ans	0-2 ans	3-5 ans	6-10 ans	0-2 ans	3-5 ans	6-10 ans	0-2 ans	3-5 ans	6-10 ans
Filles	453			44,67%			8	6,34	4,78	6	5	4
MT oui	522			51,50%								
Lieu: Urbain	573			57%								
Actes	14956	10122	10693	42%	28%	30%	14,6	9,9	10,4	12	9	9
RC totaux	10154	7402	5168	50%	60%	38%						
RC infectieux différents												
État fébrile	2160	1609	1377	26%	25%	30%	2,102	1,566	1,336			
État afébrile	1197	940	765	15%	15%	17%	1,172	0,917	0,742			
Rhino-pharyngite	2135	1321	861	26%	21%	19%	2,077	1,289	0,836			
Otite	1060	767	389	13%	12%	8%	1,028	0,751	0,378			
Angine	522	740	507	6%	12%	11%	0,511	0,724	0,496			
Bronchite	540	327	164	7%	5%	4%	0,533	0,321	0,159			
Toux	344	377	224	4%	6%	5%	0,336	0,371	0,221			
Diarrhée vomissement	249	224	266	3%	4%	6%	0,244	0,218	0,26			
4ème quartile	261	226	195	26%	22%	19%						
CM totales	431	344	302	42,50%	34%	30%						
Dermatose	210	145	141	21%	14%	14%						
Eczéma	168	96	108	17%	9%	11%						
Asthme	90	97	100	9%	10%	10%						
Rhinite	92	92	108	9%	9%	11%						

La population étudiée compte 1014 patients équitablement répartis entre les filles et les garçons. Le suivi de ces enfants sur 10 ans montre que le nombre de consultations est plus important entre 0 et 2 ans, qu'entre 3 et 5 ans ou 6 et 10 ans, avec une proportion de consultations infectieuses de plus de 50 % entre 0 et 5 ans (50% des consultations entre 0 et 2 ans, 60% entre 3 et 5 ans), puis une proportion de 38% entre 6 et 10 ans.

Les enfants âgés de 0 à 2 ans, sont ceux qui présentent le plus de comorbidités (42,5%), essentiellement dermatologiques (21%).

Il n'existe pas de différence entre les garçons et les filles concernant leur statut infectieux, sauf entre 6 et 10 ans où les filles ont une moyenne de 4,78 infections sur cette période de quatre ans, contre 4,2 pour les garçons (p=0,023). Or dans cette classe d'âge, on ne note pas de différence statistiquement significative entre les garçons et les filles en termes de comorbidités globales. La seule différence significative concerne l'asthme, atteignant plus les garçons (11,8%) que les filles (7,5 %) avec un p= 0,025. Mais cette différence est significative depuis l'âge 0-2 ans jusqu'à 6-10 ans et l'écart s'amenuise avec l'âge. Le pourcentage d'asthme est stable chez les garçons à 11,8%, tandis qu'il augmente progressivement chez les filles, passant de 5,3% entre 0 et 2 ans, à 7,3 % entre 6 et 10 ans.

Les résultats de consultation infectieux les plus fréquents sont l'état fébrile, la rhinopharyngite et l'état afébrile, ce quel que soit l'âge. Les enfants âgés de 0-2 ans sont ceux qui font le plus d'infections les plus fréquentes, avec une moyenne de 2,102 par enfant sur la période (écart type : 2,376) pour les états fébriles ; une moyenne de 2,077 par enfant sur la période (écart type : 2,482) pour les rhinopharyngites, et une moyenne de 1,172 (écart type : 1,911) pour les états afébrile. Certains enfants vont même jusqu'à faire 15 rhinopharyngites sur la période, 13 états fébriles et/ou 16 états afébriles.

Le taux de retouche pour les pathologies les plus fréquentes est faible et s'accentue avec l'âge.

Au sein des enfants faisant des infections répétées dans l'enfance (appartenant au 4ème quartile), seuls 29% restent dans le 4ème quartile jusqu'à 6-10 ans. Les autres rejoignent les quartiles moins infectés.

La moitié des enfants sont suivis par leur médecin traitant. Cette répartition est modifiée si l'on s'intéresse au lieu d'exercice des médecins. En effet, les généralistes suivent plus les enfants s'ils exercent en milieu rural et surtout semi rural qu'en milieu urbain.

V. **TYPOLOGIE :**

A. **ANALYSE EN CORRESPONDANCES MULTIPLES :**

Le traitement a lieu sur 1014 patients nés entre 1999 et 2001 et suivis de 0 à 10 ans.

Nous détaillerons ici les 5 axes principaux.

Par convention nous utiliserons les termes suivants pour définir le niveau d'infection :

Peu (1er quartile), modéré (2ème), très (3ème) et hautement (4ème).

L'axe 1 oppose les enfants très et hautement infectés quel que soit leur âge et présentant des comorbidités à tout âge, à des enfants contractant peu d'infections quel que soit leur âge et n'ayant pas de comorbidités.

L'axe 2 oppose les enfants peu infectés et sans comorbidités entre 0 et 2 ans puis hautement infectés entre 3 et 5 ans et 6 et 10 ans avec des comorbidités entre 6 et 10 ans, à des enfants modérément ou très infectés quel que soit l'âge, avec des comorbidités entre 0 et 2 ans et sans comorbidités entre 6 et 10 ans.

L'axe 3 oppose les enfants très infectés avec des comorbidités entre 0 et 2 ans puis peu infectés entre 3 et 5 ans et entre 6 et 10 ans, sans comorbidités entre 6 et 10 ans, à des enfants faiblement ou modérément infectés et sans comorbidités entre 0 et 2 ans puis modérément infectés entre 3 et 5 ans, puis très infectés avec des comorbidités entre 6 et 10 ans.

L'axe 4 oppose des enfants moyennement et très infectés et sans comorbidités entre 0 et 2 ans devenant très infectés entre 3 et 5 ans puis entre 6 et 10 ans, avec comorbidités entre 6 et 10 ans, à des enfants très infectés avec des comorbidités entre 0 et 2 ans, devenant modérément infectés entre 3 et 5 ans puis entre 6 et 10 ans, sans comorbidités entre 6 et 10 ans.

L'axe 5 oppose des enfants très infectés et sans comorbidités quel que soit l'âge, à des enfants modérément infectés avec des comorbidités quel que soit l'âge.

B. **CLASSIFICATION ASCENDANTE HIERARCHIQUE :**

La classification ascendante hiérarchique était réalisée à partir des axes représentant 80% de l'inertie de base et proposant une répartition en six, sept ou neuf classes. Nous avons choisi la répartition en sept classes résumée dans les tableaux 25, 26 et 27.

Ont été retirés du tableau les infections « pneumopathies » et « sinusites » et les comorbidités « RGO » et « carence martiale » car aucune de ces variables ne ressortaient dans la typologie quel que soit la classe d'âge.

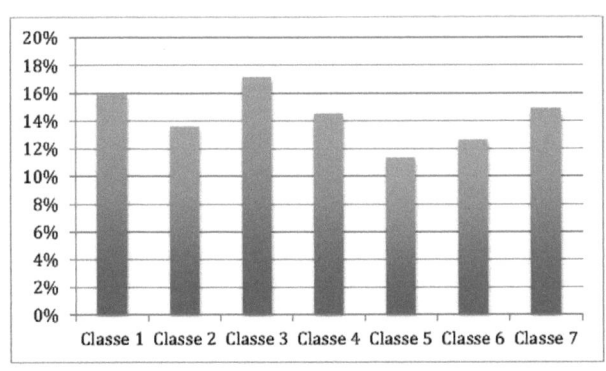

Figure 6: Pourcentage d'enfants par classes de la typologie.

Tableau 25 : Tableau récapitulatif des classes 1 et 2 de la typologie. (Variables actives soulignées)

Classes	Classe 1			Classe 2		
Titre	Peu infectés sans comorbidités quel que soit l'âge			0-2 ans modérément infectés sans comorbidités dont la moitié évoluent favorablement		
N=1014	N1=161 (15,88%)			N2= 138 (13,61%)		
Tranches d'âge	0-2 ans	3-5 ans	6-10 ans	0-2 ans	3-5 ans	6-10 ans
Nombre de RC infectieux	0-2 (58,61%)	0-2 (58,61%)	0-1 (32,21%)	3-6 (54,33%)	0-2 (28,17%) et 6-9 (20%)	0-1 (19,13%) et 2-4 (17,29%)
Commune	Urbain (72,67%)			-		
Genre	-			Filles (54,35%)		
MT	14,29%			-		
Comorbidités	Non (24,53%)	Non (20,75%)	Non (19,24%)	Non (16,64%)	Non (15,22%)	Non (15,59%)
Asthme	-	-	-	-	-	-
Dermatose	-	-	-	-	-	-
Eczéma	-	-	-	-	-	-
Rhinite	-	-	-	-	-	-
RGO	-	-	-	-	-	-
Carence martiale	-	-	-	-	-	-
RC infectieux différents	0-2 (99,38%)	0-2 (93,79%)	0-1 (63,35%) et 2-4 (31,68%)	3-5 (60,87%)	0-2 (60,14%)	0-1 (44,93%)
Angine	-	-	-	-	-	-
Bronchite	-	-	-	-	-	-
Diarrhée vomissements	-	-	-	-	-	-
État afébrile	-	-	-	37,68%	33,33%	27,54%
État fébrile	-	-	33,54%	-	52,17%	-
Otite	-	-	-	34,06%	26,09%	-
Rhinopharyngite	27,33%	-	27,33%	-	48,41	29,71
Toux	-	-	-	-	-	-

La classe 1 représente 15,88% des enfants et regroupe des enfants, sans comorbidités, peu infectés quel que soit l'âge, avec un nombre très faible de résultats de consultation infectieux différents (entre 0 et 2 quel que soit l'âge). Ils sont issus pour 72,67% d'entre eux d'un milieu urbain, et 85,71% ne sont pas suivis par leurs généralistes.

La classe 2 représente 13,61% des enfants. Il s'agit d'enfants modérément infectés entre 0 et 2 ans dont environ la moitié, évoluent favorablement en étant peu infectés entre 3 et 10 ans. L'autre moitié quant à elle, reste modérément infectée. Ils ne présentent aucune comorbidité quel que soit l'âge et le nombre de RC infectieux différents est important entre 0 et 2 ans et diminue avec l'âge. Ils contractent les pathologies les plus fréquemment retrouvées en pédiatrie de ville (états fébriles : 30% en moyenne ; rhinopharyngites : 48,41% entre 3 et 5 ans et 29,71% entre 6 et 10 ans ; états afébriles : 52,17% entre 3 et 5 ans) mais également des pathologies ORL (otites : 30% en moyenne entre 0 et 2 ans). Cette classe est constituée d'une prédominance de filles (54,35%), ce qui représente 16,56% des filles de l'échantillon. Il s'agit de la seule classe où une différence entre les filles et les garçons est mise en évidence.

Tableau 26 : Tableau récapitulatif des classes 3, 4 et 5 de la typologie.

Classes	Classe 3			Classe 4			Classe 5		
Titre	3-5 ans modérément infectés sans comorbidités			0-2 ans très infectés évoluant favorablement avec l'âge			0-2 ans hautement infectés évoluant favorablement avec l'âge		
N=1014	N3= 174 (17,16%)			N4= 147 (14,50%)			N5= 115 (11,34%)		
Tranches d'âge	0-2 ans	3-5 ans	6-10 ans	0-2 ans	3-5 ans	6-10 ans	0-2 ans	3-5 ans	6-10 ans
Nombre de RC infectieux	0-2 (22,34%) et 3-6 (28,74%)	3-5 (69,88%)	>7 (9,74%)	7-11 (65,04%)	6-9 (25,88%)	0-1 (19,13%)	>11 (42,53%)	6-9 (19,22%)	2-4 (30,17%)
Commune	-			-			Semi Rural (43,48%) et Urbain (40,87%)		
Genre	-			-			-		
MT	39,66%			66,67%			80%		
Co-morbidités	Non (24,53%)	Non (20,45%)	-	Oui (22,97%)	-	Non (16,57%)	Oui (19,03%)	Oui (14,83%)	-
Asthme	-	-	-	-	-	-	-	-	-
Dermatose	-	-	-	35,37%	-	-	38,26%	-	-
Eczéma	-	-	-	-	-	-	30,43%	-	-
Rhinite	-	-	-	-	-	-	-	-	-
RGO	-	-	-	-	-	-	-	-	-
Carence martiale	-	-	-	-	-	-	-	-	-
RC infectieux différents	0-2 (50%)	3-4 (61,49%)	0-1 (42,53%)	3-5 (87,76%)	-	0-1 (44,90%)	>5 (45,22%)	3-4 (57,39%)	2-4 (69,57%)
Angine	-	-	-	-	-	-	50,43%	-	-
Bronchite	-	-	-	42,18%	-	-	54,78%	-	-
Diarrhée vomissements	-	-	-	-	-	-	38,26%	-	-
État afébrile	35,06%	33,33%	27,59%	61,90%	-	-	80,87%	56,52%	-
État fébrile	58,05%	-	50,57%	89,12%	76,87%	29,93%	97,39%	81,74%	-
Otite	34,48%	-	-	-	-	-	78,26%	53,04%	-
Rhinopharyngite	55,75%	-	-	86,39%	-	31,97%	87,83%	-	-
Toux	-	-	-	31,97%	-	-	40,87%	-	-

La classe 3 est la plus importante et représente 17,16% des enfants. Il s'agit d'enfants peu à modérément infectés entre 0 et 5 ans, sans comorbidités, avec des RC infectieux différents peu nombreux (0 à 2 entre 0 et 2 ans puis 3 à 4 entre 3 et 5 ans). Ils présentent les infections les plus fréquemment retrouvées (états fébrile : 30% en moyenne ; rhinopharyngites : 55,75% entre 0 et 2 ans, états fébriles : 58,05% entre 0 et 2 ans) et des infections ORL (otites : 34,4% entre 0 et 2 ans). Puis ces enfants deviennent très infectés entre 6 et 10 ans (plus de 7 RC infectieux), et font essentiellement les infections les plus fréquentes (états fébriles : 50,57% et états afébriles : 27,59%). Ils sont suivis essentiellement par quelqu'un d'autre que leur généraliste (60,34%).

La classe 4 représente 14,50% des enfants. Il s'agit d'enfants très infectés entre 0 et 2 ans, avec des comorbidités (35,37% de ces enfants ont des dermatoses), très infectés entre 3 et 5 ans, puis peu infectés entre 6 et 10 ans, sans comorbidités. Ils font un nombre important de RC infectieux différents entre 0 et 2 ans puis le nombre de RC infectieux différents devient très faible entre 6 et 10 ans (44,90% entre 0 et 1). Ils présentent les infections les plus fréquentes (états fébriles : 89,12% entre 0 et 2 ans, 76,87% entre 3 et 5 ans et 29,93% entre 6 et 10 ans ; rhinopharyngites: 86,39% entre 0 et 2 ans et 31,97% entre 6 et 10 ans ; états afébriles : 61,90% entre 0 et 2 ans) ; mais aussi des infections des voies aériennes inférieures (bronchites : 42,18% entre 0 et 2 ans ; toux : 31,97% entre 0 et 2 ans) ; sans infections ORL : otite et angine), Ces enfants sont suivis pour 66.67% d'entre eux par leur généraliste et 25.85% d'entre eux sont en milieu rural.

La classe 5 représente 11,34% des enfants. Elle regroupe 42,53% des enfants hautement infectés entre 0 et 2 ans (supérieur à 11 RC) avec des comorbidités entre 0 et 2 ans (essentiellement de l'eczéma et des dermatoses) Ils font un nombre très important de RC infectieux différents quel que soit leur âge, surtout entre 0 et 2 ans. Ils présentent les infections les plus fréquentes (états fébriles : 97,39% entre 0 et 2 ans et 81,74% entre 3 et 5 ans; rhinopharyngites : 87,83% entre 0 et 2 ans ; états afébriles : 80,87% entre 0 et 2 ans et 56,52% entre 3 et 5 ans) ; des infections ORL (otites : 78,26% entre 0 et 2 ans et 53,04% entre 3 et 5 ans ; angines : 50,43% entre 0 et 2 ans) mais aussi des pathologies digestives (diarrhée vomissements : 38,26% entre 0 et 2 ans). Ces enfants sont de moins en moins infectés avec l'âge (6 à 9 RC entre 3 et 5 ans, puis 2 à 4 RC entre 6 et 10 ans). Il s'agit essentiellement d'enfants issus de milieux semi-ruraux (43,48%) et urbains (40,87%), suivis pour 80% d'entre eux par leurs généralistes.

Tableau 27 : Tableau récapitulatif des classes 6 et 7 de la typologie.

Classes	Classe 6			Classe 7		
Titre	Hautement infectés en 3-5 ans, très infectés en 0-2 et 6-10 ans, avec 1/5ème de comorbidités			Hautement infectés quel que soit l'âge avec comorbidités		
N=1014	N6= 128 (12,62%)			N7= 151 (14,89%)		
Classes d'âge	0-2 ans	3-5 ans	6-10 ans	0-2 ans	3-5 ans	6-10 ans
Nombre de RC infectieux	>11 (22,61%)	6-9 (16,86%) et >9 (30,09%)	5-7 (56,64%)	>11 (28,35%)	>9 (45,13%)	>7 (76,92%)
Commune	-			Semi Rural (33,77%) et Urbain (48,34%)		
Genre	-			-		
MT	-			65,56%		
Comorbidités	Oui (15,55%)	Oui (19,77%)	Oui (18,87%)	Oui (21,58%)	Oui (24,42%)	Oui (31,13%)
Asthme	-	-	-	-	-	29,14%
Dermatose	-	-	-	31,13%	-	-
Eczéma	-	-	-	-	-	-
Rhinite	-	-	-	74,83%	-	-
RGO	-	-	-	-	-	-
Carence martiale	-	-	-	-	-	-
RC infectieux différents	0-2 (27,34%)	3-4 (49,22%) et >4 (42,19%)	2-4 (80,47%)	-	>4 (60,26%)	>4 (53,64%)
Angine	-	53,91%	47,66%	48,34%	61,59%	56,29%
Bronchite	-	-	-	37,09%	40,40%	29,14%
Diarrhée vomissements	-	-	-		36,42%	39,74%
État afébrile	-	60,94%	62,50%	60,26%	66,23%	71,52%
État fébrile	-	85,16%	86,72%	78,81%	84,77%	92,05%
Otite	53,91%	60,94%	35,16%	55,63%	62,26%	49,01%
Rhinopharyngite	75%	72,66%	54,69%		80,79%	80,79%
Toux	-	32,81%	-	35, 76%	43,05%	38,41%

La classe 6 représente 12,62% des enfants. Elle regroupe des enfants hautement infectés entre 0 et 5 ans puis très infectés entre 6 et 10 ans, dont environ 1/5ème ont des comorbidités quel que soit l'âge. On retrouve les pathologies les plus fréquentes (rhinopharyngites : 75% entre 0 et 2 ans, 72,66% entre 3 e 5 ans et 54,69% entre 6 et 10 ans ; états fébriles : 85,16% entre 3 et 5 ans et 86,72% entre 6 et 10 ans ; états afébriles : environ 60% entre 3 et 10 ans) mais également des pathologies ORL (angines : 50% en moyenne entre 3 et 10 ans; otites : 53,91% entre 0 et 2 ans, 60,94% entre 3 et 5 ans et 35,16% entre 6 et 10 ans). Le nombre de RC infectieux différents augmente avec l'âge, puisque 80,47% des enfants de cette classe font entre 2 et 4 RC infectieux différents entre 6 et 10 ans.

La classe 7 regroupe 14,89% des enfants. Il s'agit d'enfants très infectés avec des comorbidités quel que soit leur âge (rhinites et dermatoses entre 0 et 2 ans puis asthme entre 6 et 10 ans). Ils font tous types d'infections en grandes proportions avec les pathologies les plus fréquentes (états afébriles : 65% en moyenne ; rhinopharyngites : 80,79% entre 3 et 10 ans ; états fébriles : 85% en moyenne), les infections ORL (angines : 55% en moyenne ; otites : 55% en moyenne), les infections des voies aériennes inférieures (bronchite : entre 30 et 40% ; toux : 40% en moyenne) et les infections digestives (diarrhée vomissements : 37% en moyenne entre 3 et 10 ans). Ils ont un nombre de RC infectieux différents très importants surtout entre 3 et 10 ans (supérieur à 4 RC) et 25% en moyenne tout âge confondu, ont des comorbidités. Il s'agit d'enfants issus des milieux urbains (48,34%) et semi-ruraux (33,77%), suivis pour 65,56% d'entre eux par leurs généralistes.

VI. ANALYSE DES TRAITEMENTS PAR ANTIBIOTIQUES :

A. ANALYSE DESCRIPTIVE

Tableau 28: Pourcentage de prescription d'antibiotiques en fonction du type de pathologies diagnostiquées

Résultats de consultation	Prescription totale d'antibiotique pour le RC	Prescription d'antibiotiques si le RC infectieux est seul	Prescription d'antibiotiques si le RC infectieux est associé à un autre RC infectieux.
SINUSITE	76%	75%	100%
OTITE MOYENNE	71%	66%	78%
ANGINE (AMYGDALITE - PHARYNGITE)	69%	67%	83%
BRONCHITE AIGUË	63%	58%	77%
PNEUMOPATHIE AIGUE	58%	57%	69%
RHINOPHARYNGITE - RHUME	34%	27%	73%
ETAT FEBRILE	26%	23%	69%
ETAT MORBIDE AFEBRILE	18%	15%	56%
TOUX	15%	10%	47%
DIARRHEE NAUSEE VOMISSEMENT	4%	2%	35%

Le tableau ci-dessus montre le pourcentage de prescription d'antibiotiques en fonction du type de pathologies diagnostiquées. On remarque qu'il y a deux groupes d'infections : un groupe d'infections traitées par antibiotique dans 60 à 75% des cas, constituées des sinusites, des otites moyennes, des angines, des bronchites et des pneumopathies, et un groupe d'infections traitées par antibiotiques dans 1/3 des cas, regroupant les rhinopharyngites, les états fébriles, les états afébriles, les toux et les diarrhées vomissements.

Dans ce deuxième groupe d'infections, en cas d'association avec un autre RC infectieux, la prescription d'antibiotique est multipliée par un facteur 3 pour la rhinopharyngite et l'état fébrile, un facteur 4 pour l'état afébrile, un facteur 5 pour la toux et un facteur 17 pour les diarrhées vomissements.

B. ANALYSE PAR CLASSES DE LA TYPOLOGIE :

1. Par prescription d'antibiotiques :

Figure 7: Répartition des antibiotiques prescrits en pourcentage, par classes de la typologie.

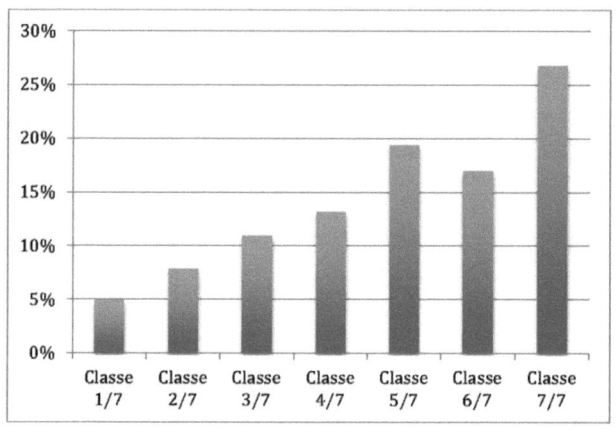

Les classes de la typologie pour lesquelles les patients sont très (classe 6) ou hautement (classe 7) infectés, et hautement infectés entre 0 et 2 ans (classe 5) sont celles qui reçoivent le plus d'antibiotiques.

Tableau 29: Nombre d'antibiotiques (AB) prescrits par classe de la typologie et par classes d'âge.

Nombre d'AB prescrits	0-2 ans	3-5 ans	6-10 ans	Total	Nombre d'AB prescrits	0-2 ans	3-5 ans	6-10 ans	Total
Classe 1/7	52	74	289	415	Classe 1/7	1%	3%	12%	5%
Classe 2/7	219	171	270	660	Classe 2/7	6%	7%	11%	8%
Classe 3/7	324	233	361	918	Classe 3/7	9%	10%	15%	11%
Classe 4/7	521	294	287	1102	Classe 4/7	15%	12%	12%	13%
Classe 5/7	1048	353	227	1628	Classe 5/7	30%	15%	9%	19%
Classe 6/7	588	476	361	1425	Classe 6/7	17%	20%	15%	17%
Classe 7/7	789	765	692	2246	Classe 7/7	22%	32%	28%	27%
Total général	3541	2366	2487	8394	Total général	100%	100%	100%	100%

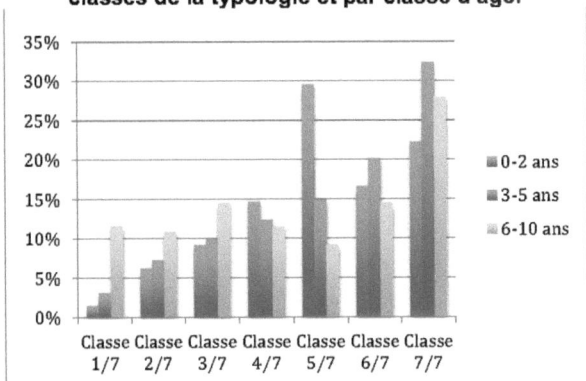

Figure 8: Pourcentage d'antibiotiques prescrits par classes de la typologie et par classe d'âge.

On remarque qu'il y a trois types de prescriptions d'antibiotiques.

Un premier type concernant les classes 1, 2 et 3, où la prescription augmente avec l'âge, et nettement pour les 6-10 ans. Pour mémoire, les classes 1 et 2 regroupent des enfants peu ou modérément infectés quel que soit l'âge. La classe 3 regroupe des enfants modérément infectés entre 3 et 5 ans, sans comorbidités.

Un second type concernant les classes 4 et 5, où la prescription décroît avec l'âge. Pour mémoire, les classes 4 et 5 sont les enfants hautement ou très infectés entre 0 et 2 ans, évoluant favorablement.

Un troisième type concernant les classes 6 et 7, où les 3-5 ans reçoivent le plus d'antibiotiques, avec des prescriptions qui restent élevées pour la classe 7. Pour mémoire, les classes 6 et 7 regroupent des enfants très ou hautement infectés quel que soit l'âge.

2. Par nombre de patients recevant des antibiotiques :

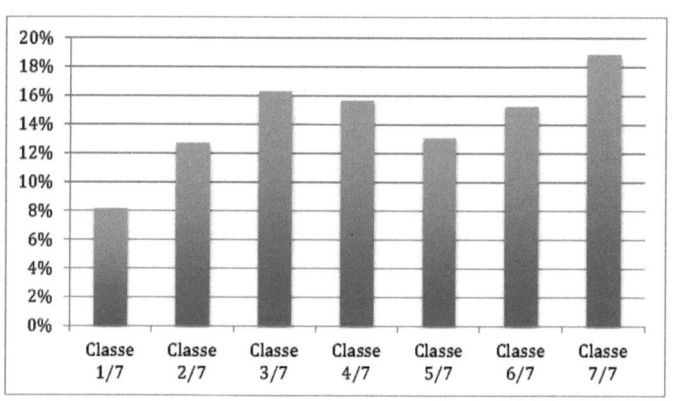

Figure 9: Nombre de patients par classes de la typologie, recevant des antibiotiques.

Au sein de chaque classe, moins de 20% des patients reçoivent des antibiotiques.

Tableau 30: Nombre de patients recevant des antibiotiques par classes de la typologie et par classes d'âge (en valeurs absolues et en pourcentages)

Nombre de patients recevant des antibiotiques	0-2 ans	3-5 ans	6-10 ans	Total	Nombre de patients recevant des antibiotiques	0-2 ans	3-5 ans	6-10 ans	Total
Classe 1/7	43	40	93	176	Classe 1/7	6%	6%	12%	8%
Classe 2/7	107	68	99	274	Classe 2/7	15%	10%	13%	13%
Classe 3/7	108	116	128	352	Classe 3/7	15%	17%	17%	16%
Classe 4/7	129	102	108	339	Classe 4/7	18%	15%	14%	16%
Classe 5/7	107	96	79	282	Classe 5/7	15%	14%	10%	13%
Classe 6/7	112	112	106	330	Classe 6/7	15%	17%	14%	15%
Classe 7/7	125	142	141	408	Classe 7/7	17%	21%	19%	19%
Total général	731	676	754	2161	Total général	100%	100%	100%	100%

Figure 10: Nombre de patients recevant des antibiotiques par classe de la typologie et par classes d'âge.

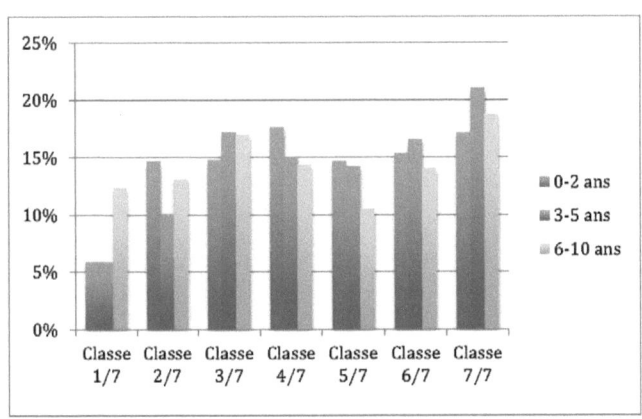

Concernant le nombre de patients par classe de la typologie recevant des antibiotiques, on remarque qu'il y a deux extrêmes, à savoir les enfants de la classe 1, dont 8% reçoivent des antibiotiques, et les enfants de la classe 7, dont 19% reçoivent des antibiotiques. Le nombre d'enfants par classe recevant des antibiotiques fluctue entre 13 et 16 % pour les classes 2, 3, 4, 5 et 6.

VII. CHOIX DE LA CLASSE PERMETTANT DE REPÉRER LES ENFANTS LES PLUS INFECTÉS :

La typologie met en évidence deux classes hautement (classe 7) ou très infectées (classe 6). Afin de repérer au mieux les enfants les plus infectés, nous avons testé une sélection d'une part sur la classe 7 et d'autre part sur les classes 6 et 7, et avons réalisé les courbes ROC suivantes.

Figure 11 : Courbe ROC de la classe 7.

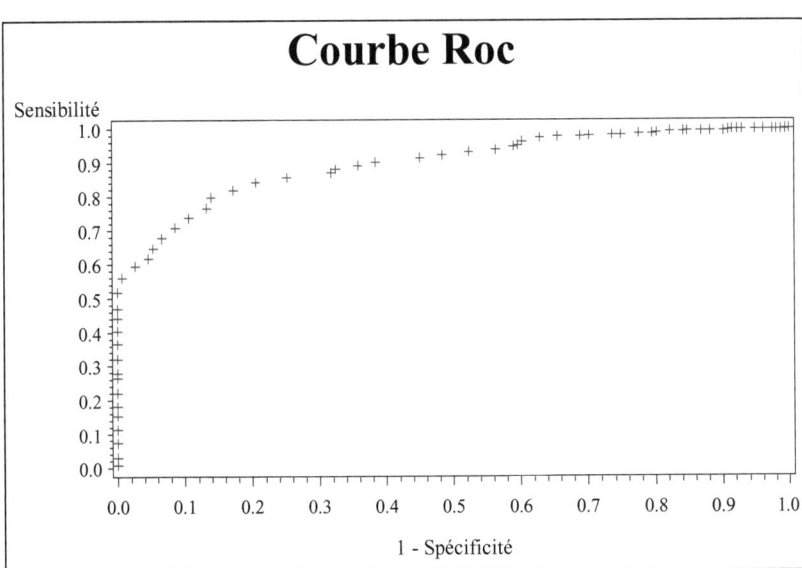

Figure 12: Courbe ROC des classes 6 et 7.

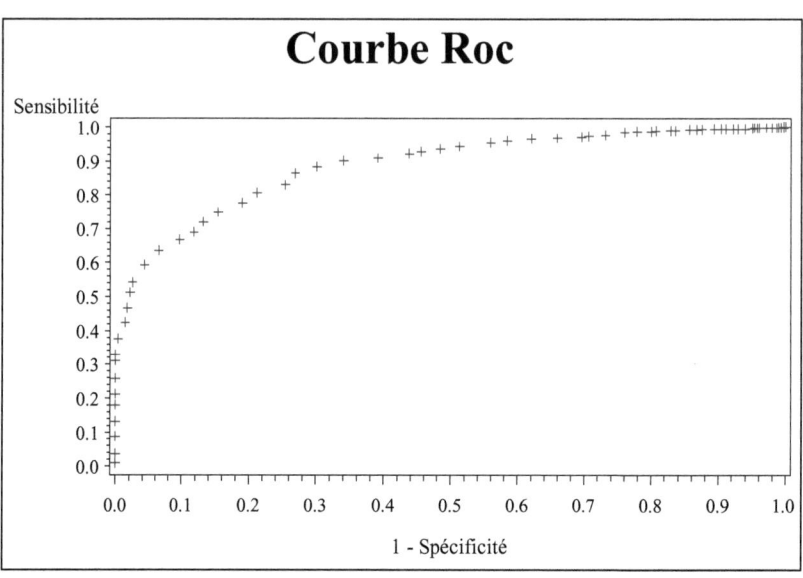

L'aire sous la courbe de la classe 7 semble meilleure que celle des classes 6 et 7. De plus avec la sélection de la classe 7, on obtient une sensibilité à 84,2% et une spécificité à 79,5%, ce qui nous permet de ne sélectionner que 120 patients. Avec la sélection des classes 6 et 7, on obtient une sensibilité à 83% et une spécificité à 74,6%, en sélectionnant 208 patients.

Ainsi nous avons sélectionné la classe 7 car suffisamment précise pour repérer les enfants les plus infectés.

VIII. DISCUSSION :

L'originalité de ce travail se situe en premier lieu dans la vision globale qu'il apporte sur les infections dites à répétition de l'enfant. En effet, la bibliographie faite pour réaliser ce travail montre que les études sur le sujet s'intéressent le plus souvent à un type précis de pathologie (otites, rhinopharyngites, bronchites ou bronchiolites, etc.). Seules trois études(8)(9)(12) s'intéressent à l'ensemble du statut infectieux de l'enfant, toutes pathologies confondues.

De même beaucoup d'études travaillent sur les enfants âgés de 0 à 2 ans (âge préscolaire), se questionnant notamment sur l'impact du mode de garde sur la fréquence des infections de l'enfant, mais très peu s'intéressent aux enfants âgés de 3-5 ans (maternelle) et 6-10 ans (primaires).

Un autre atout de cette étude est l'importance de l'échantillon sur lequel nous avons travaillé (1014 enfants). Les études sur le sujet présentent des échantillons nettement plus faibles variant entre 100 et 498 patients (3)(4)(10)(13)(18)(26)(31).

Enfin, dans la littérature, aucune typologie sur le statut infectieux des enfants en médecine générale n'a été retrouvée.

L'étude réalisée montre que les principaux problèmes posés par les enfants en médecine générale concernent des problèmes infectieux dans plus de 50% des cas entre 0 et 5 ans, et dans 40% des cas entre 6 et 10 ans, toutes pathologies confondues. Cela justifie donc le fait que l'on s'y intéresse.

Cependant, il est intéressant de noter, que seuls 27,5% de ces enfants restent très ou hautement infectés entre 0 et 10 ans.

De la typologie en 7 classes, assez détaillée, que nous avons réalisé au cours de cette étude, nous pouvons retenir, pour le clinicien, un résumé en trois groupes.

Un premier groupe très peu infecté quel que soit l'âge (classe 1) représentant 15,88% des enfants étudiés. Cela signifie qu'ils sont vus, pour des problèmes infectieux, maximum une fois par an entre 0 et 2 ans, puis une fois tous les ans et demi entre 3 et 5 ans, puis une fois tous les deux ans et demi entre 6 et 10 ans. Ils ont un nombre de résultats de consultation infectieux différents très faible et sont vus essentiellement pour des rhinopharyngites et des états fébriles. Ils ne présentent pas de comorbidités.

Un deuxième groupe est hautement ou très infectés quel que soit l'âge (classes 6 et 7) et regroupe 27,51% des enfants étudiés. Ces enfants sont vus pour des problèmes infectieux, minimum une fois tous les deux mois entre 0 et 2 ans, puis une fois tous les quatre à six mois entre 3 et 5 ans, puis une fois par an à une fois tous les huit mois et demi entre 6 et 10 ans.

Ils ont un nombre de résultats de consultation infectieux différents important et font tous types de pathologies infectieuses. Ils présentent des comorbidités.

Et enfin un troisième groupe, intermédiaire (classes 2, 3, 4 et 5) représentant 56,61% des enfants. Ils ont un nombre de résultats de consultation infectieux différents intermédiaire (2 à 4), qui est le plus élevé entre 0 et 2 ans.

Concernant le médecin traitant, on remarque que les classes pour lesquelles le médecin traitant n'est pas majoritaire sont les classes avec les enfants les moins infectés avec absence de comorbidités. En réalité on ne peut connaitre le statut infectieux exact de ces enfants, puisqu'on peut penser qu'ils ne consultent pas régulièrement le médecin de notre échantillon.

La cible par rapport à l'objectif de notre travail, concernait à priori les enfants des classes 6 et 7, soit un peu moins d'un tiers des enfants. La classe 7 est hautement infectée (4ème quartile) de 0 à 10 ans et la classe 6 hautement infectée entre 0 et 2 ans puis très infectée (3ème quartile) entre 3 et 10 ans. La question était de savoir si l'on choisissait plutôt la classe 7 ou les classes 6 et

7 pour le repérage des enfants à risque d'infections à répétition. L'apport de la classe 6 n'améliorait pas la sensibilité et spécificité ce qui nous a amené à choisir la classe 7 et donc de centrer les efforts de dépistage sur 12% des enfants (Se= 84%, Spe=79,5%).

Au regard de ces éléments on voit donc se dessiner le profil de l'enfant à risque d'infections répétées : il s'agit d'un enfant hautement infecté dès 0-2 ans, avec une consultation pour des problèmes infectieux une fois tous les 2 mois, présentant des comorbidités de type de rhinites et/ou de dermatoses, issu d'un milieu urbain ou semi-rural et faisant tous type d'infections (dont une proportion d'infections ORL plus importante (55%) que les autres enfants) pour lesquelles le recours aux antibiotiques est fréquent. On voit également que parmi ces enfants très infectés entre 0 et 2 ans, seuls 28,35% le restent entre 3 et 5 ans puis entre 6 et 10 ans. Il est donc difficile de repérer de façon évidente, dès 0-2 ans, les enfants qui vont poser ou pas des problèmes, liés à ces infections répétées.

Ainsi, le repérage d'un enfant très régulièrement infecté avec les variables disponibles pour notre étude, est possible : il s'agit d'un enfant issu d'un milieu urbain ou semi rural, faisant plus de 11 infections de tout type, sur la période de 0 à 2 ans, (états fébriles, états afébriles, otites, angines, bronchites, toux), et présentant des comorbidités de type rhinites et/ou dermatoses. Cet enfant fait plus de 9 infections, de tout type sur la période de 3 à 5 ans (états fébriles, rhinopharyngites, états afébriles, otites, angines, toux, bronchites, diarrhées vomissements), avec plus de 4 résultats de consultation différents sur cette même période. Enfin, cet enfant se différencie réellement des autres à partir de la période 6-10 ans, car il continue à faire un grand nombre d'infections, plus de 7 sur la période, de tout type (états fébriles, rhinopharyngites, états afébriles, angines, otites, diarrhées vomissements, toux, bronchites), avec un nombre de résultats de consultation différents supérieur à 4 sur cette même période. Il présente également des comorbidités à type d'asthme entre 6 et 10 ans.

Au sein de ce travail, certains éléments confirment ce qui avait déjà été trouvé au cours de précédentes études. L'activité du généraliste auprès des nourrissons et des enfants de 3 à 10 ans est, pour une grande partie, en rapport avec les pathologies infectieuses, avec 50% chez les 0-2 ans (Élisabeth Griot(1) retrouvait 45,7% en 1995), et 49% entre 3 et 10 ans (52,9% en 1995). De plus comme le souligne Robert Cohen(4) en 2005, il est normal de faire plusieurs infections respiratoires dans les premières années de vie, cependant pour lui *« six à dix épisodes de rhinopharyngites sont la règle dans les premières années de vie, le pic de fréquence se situant entre six et 18 mois »*, or dans notre étude seuls 17% des enfants âgés de 0 et 2 ans font six à huit rhinopharyngites, la moyenne sur cette période étant de 2,077 (écart type : 2,482).

Cette différence de résultats peut être due à une différence de définition du terme rhinopharyngite entre les deux études, étant donné la richesse et la précision du dictionnaire des résultats de consultation. En effet, sur cette période nous avons aussi recensé 14,5% d'enfants faisant entre six à huit états fébriles et 14% d'enfants faisant entre six à huit états afébriles.

Concernant les définitions des infections à répétition retrouvées dans le cadre du dépistage des déficits immunitaires, nos résultats renforcent ce qui avait été trouvé précédemment:

- Otites récidivantes : trois épisodes en six mois ou quatre épisodes en un an. (14). Cela reviendrait à dire, plus de 8 otites entre 0 et 2 ans ou entre 3 et 5 ans, ce qui correspond dans notre étude à 17 enfants entre 0 et 2 ans soit 1,6% des enfants étudiés, et 2 enfants entre 3 et 5 ans soit 0,2% des enfants étudiés. Cette définition paraît donc très discriminante.

- Angines récidivantes: sept ou plus en une année ou dix durant les deux à trois dernières années (15). Dans notre étude, aucun enfant ne

présente de telle caractéristiques, cette définition est donc également très discriminante.
- Rhinopharyngites : plus de six épisodes de rhinopharyngites fébriles par an après l'âge de trois ans (4). Dans notre étude, aucun enfant ne présente de telle caractéristiques, cette définition est donc également très discriminante.
- D'après Siegrist, une infection pulmonaire mérite qu'on y prête une attention particulière car plus suspecte d'un déficit sous-jacent(21). Cette notion est retrouvée dans notre typologie, car la pneumopathie a une fréquence infime au sein de notre population.

Ainsi la problématique dysimmunitaire est une problématique infime pour un médecin généraliste.

Une donnée intéressante retrouvée par McCutcheon « montre que les enfants qui n'ont pas fréquenté de crèche sont plus souvent malades à un âge scolaire que les enfants mis en collectivité à un âge précoce »(35). Ce groupe d'enfants pourrait être représenté par la classe 3 de notre typologie, regroupant, rappelons-le, des enfants peu ou modérément infectés entre 0 et 2 ans, qui deviennent de plus en plus infectés avec l'âge.

Certains facteurs individuels retrouvés dans la littérature comme favorisant la répétition des infections étudiées, sont également mis en évidence dans notre étude, tels que :
- l'âge précoce de début des premiers épisodes(6) : les enfants des classes 6 et 7 de notre typologie, sont hautement infectés dès 0-2 ans.
- l'asthme(7) : les enfants de la classe 7, présente pour 29,14% d'entre eux, un asthme entre 6 et 10 ans.

En revanche certains autres éléments ne sont pas retrouvés :
- la carence martiale, le RGO et le sexe masculin(6) : dans notre typologie, les comorbidités carence martiale et RGO ne ressortent nulle part et les filles sont plus sujettes aux infections entre 6 et 10 ans que les garçons sans explication retrouvée (possible effet lié à notre échantillon).

Concernant la prescription d'antibiotiques, on sait que la France est un des plus gros prescripteur et qu'il existe une variabilité de prescription en fonction des médecins(36)(37)(48)(49).

Notre étude suggère qu'il existe aussi 3 attitudes de prescriptions des médecins, celles-ci pouvant s'intriquer:
- en fonction des pathologies : si l'étiologie peut être bactérienne, on note une plus grande prescription d'antibiotique que si l'étiologie est virale.
- si plusieurs résultats de consultation infectieux sont associés, le risque de prescription d'antibiotiques est plus élevé.
- la typologie nous montre que les classes où les enfants les plus infectées sont les plus traitées par antibiotiques.

Ceci étant le nombre d'enfants qui reçoivent des antibiotiques par classes est inférieur à 20 %. On peut émettre l'hypothèse qu'il s'agit donc toujours des mêmes enfants qui reçoivent des antibiotiques et que les enfants ayant déjà reçu des antibiotiques sont plus à risque d'en recevoir à nouveau.

Les limites de notre étude sont :
- L'utilisation de données issues d'un réseau de médecins généralistes volontaires et informatisés.

- Le fait que nous n'avons pu travailler que sur des données cliniques enregistrées en continue.
- Le manque d'un certain nombre de données telles que des données contextuelles et socio-professionnelles, du mode de garde des enfants, de l'existence ou non d'une fratrie et la place au sein de celle-ci, de la présence ou non d'animaux domestiques au domicile, des antécédents néonataux et familiaux. En réalité ces données ne sont jamais recueillies en continue par les médecins.

IX. **CONCLUSION :**

A l'issue de notre étude nous pouvons dire que 15% des enfants méritent une attention particulière quant à leurs infections à répétition. Le médecin généraliste peut repérer ces enfants de la manière suivante : surveillance particulière des enfants faisant plus de six infections par an entre 0 et 2 ans et plus de cinq infections par an entre 3 et 5 ans. Entre 6-10 ans, ces enfants continuent à faire des infections à répétition (plus de 2 infections par an) de type très varié et présentent des comorbidités notamment de type asthme.

Une des conséquences directes pour ces enfants est le risque de recevoir plus d'antibiotiques que les autres enfants, réponse thérapeutique inappropriée pour résoudre cette problématique d'infections à répétition.

La question des déterminants notamment sociaux et contextuels, susceptibles d'expliquer ces infections à répétition reste ouverte et devra faire l'objet d'une prochaine étude pour compléter ce travail.

X. BIBLIOGRAPHIE :

1. GRIOT E. LES CONSULTATIONS D'ENFANTS EN MEDECINE GENERALE. CONSOMMATION MEDICALE, AFFECTIONS PEDIATRIQUES EN SOINS PRIMAIRES [Internet]. 1995.

2. Mahlaoui N. Explorations immunitaires chez l'enfant suivi pour infections respiratoires récurrentes. Immune explorations on children suffering from recurrent respiratory tract infections. Archives de pédiatrie. 2007;

3. Jesenak M, Majtan J, Rennerova Z, Kyselovic J, Banovcin P, Hrubisko M. Immunomodulatory effect of pleuran (β-glucan from Pleurotus ostreatus) in children with recurrent respiratory tract infections. Int Immunopharmacol [Internet]. 19 déc 2012.

4. Cohen R, Just J, Koskas M, Bingen E, Boucherat M, Bourrillon A, et al. [Recurrent respiratory tract infections: how should we investigate and treat?]. Arch Pédiatrie Organe Off Sociéte Française Pédiatrie. févr 2005;12(2):183- 190.

5. Monto AS. Studies of the community and family: acute respiratory illness and infection. Epidemiol Rev. 1994;16(2):351- 373.

6. REINERT P, STAGNARA J, ROY P, MALLET E, GAUDELUS J. Rhinopharyngites et otites à répétition de l'enfant : Infections aiguës des voies respiratoires de l'enfant. Rev Prat [Internet]. 14 avr 2008;ol. 57, n° 16, 2007, pages 1767-1773, 26 réf., ISSN 0035-2640, FRA.

7. Pósfay Barbe KM, Barazzone-Argiroffo C, Siegrist C-A. Infections récurrentes des voies respiratoires inférieures de l'enfant : quand et comment les investiguer ? Rev Médicale Suisse [Internet]. (3007).

8. SANNINO N, BELKHAYAT M. Pathologies infectieuses et mode de garde des enfants d'âge préscolaire [Internet]. Dossiers d'études. Allocations Familiales; 2002.

9. FLORET D. Incidence des infections en crèche. Comparaison des différents modes de garde. Archives de pédiatrie, 6, suppl. 3, 615-617.; 1996.

10. MONGALGI L., GUEDDANA N, ZOUARI B. Facteurs environnementaux des infections respiratoires aiguës répétées: Etude statistique Environmental risk factors for recurrent acute respiratory tract infection. A statistical study. Ann Pédiatrie Paris. 1998;Annales de pédiatrie (Paris) A. 1998, vol. 45, n° 9, pp. 665-668 [bibl. : 5 ref.](n°9, vol 45):665- 668.

11. OVETCHKINE P, COHEN R. Infections respiratoires et collectivités = Respiratory acquired community infections. Arch Pédiatrie.

12. Guedeney A, Grasso F, Starakis N. Le séjour en crèche des jeunes enfants : sécurité de l'attachement, tempérament et fréquence des maladies. Psychiatr Enfant. 2004;47(1):259.

13. COHEN R. Otites récidivantes et vaccins. Médecine Enfance [Internet]. sept 2003;

14. Bluestone C, Klein J. Otitis media in infants and children. 1995.

15. Clinical practice guideline: management of sinusitis. Pediatrics. sept 2001;108(3):798- 808.

16. Wald ER. Recurrent and nonresolving pneumonia in children. Semin Respir Infect. mars 1993;8(1):46- 58.

17. Tabachnik E, Levison H. Postgraduate course presentation. Infantile bronchial asthma. J Allergy Clin Immunol. mai 1981;67(5):339- 347.

18. Harsten G, Prellner K, Heldrup J, Kalm O, Kornfält R. Recurrent acute otitis media. A prospective study of children during the first three years of life. Acta Otolaryngol (Stockh). févr 1989;107(1-2):111- 119.

19. Benediktsdóttir B. Upper airway infections in preschool children--frequency and risk factors. Scand J Prim Health Care. sept 1993;11(3):197- 201.

20. Hardy AM, Fowler MG. Child care arrangements and repeated ear infections in young children. Am J Public Health. sept 1993;83(9):1321- 1325.

21. Siegrist CA. [The child with recurrent infections: which screening for immunoe deficiency?]. Arch Pédiatrie Organe Off Sociéte Française Pédiatrie. févr 2001;8(2):205- 210.

22. Anderson LJ, Parker RA, Strikas RA, Farrar JA, Gangarosa EJ, Keyserling HL, et al. Day-care center attendance and hospitalization for lower respiratory tract illness. Pediatrics. sept 1988;82(3):300- 308.

23. Fleming DW, Cochi SL, Hightower AW, Broome CV. Childhood upper respiratory tract infections: to what degree is incidence affected by day-care attendance? Pediatrics. janv 1987;79(1):55- 60.

24. Sennerstam RB. Absence due to illness among toddlers in day-care centres in relation to child group structure. Public Health. mars 1997;111(2):85- 88.

25. Gryczyńska D, Kobos J, Zakrzewska A. Relationship between passive smoking, recurrent respiratory tract infections and otitis media in children. Int J Pediatr Otorhinolaryngol 549 Suppl 1S275-8. oct 1999;

26. Mäntymaa M, Puura K, Luoma I, Salmelin R, Davis H, Tsiantis J, et al. Infant-mother interaction as a predictor of child's chronic health problems. Child Care Health Dev. mai 2003;29(3):181- 191.

27. DUTAU G. L'infection précoce en crèche : facteur protecteur de l'allergie ou non ? Médecine Enfance. Sptembre 2002;

28. Etzel RA, Pattishall EN, Haley NJ, Fletcher RH, Henderson FW. Passive smoking and middle ear effusion among children in day care. Pediatrics. août 1992;90(2 Pt 1):228- 232.

29. Holberg CJ, Wright AL, Martinez FD, Morgan WJ, Taussig LM. Child day care, smoking by caregivers, and lower respiratory tract illness in the first 3 years of life. Group Health Medical Associates. Pediatrics. mai 1993;91(5):885- 892.

30. Celedon JC, Litonjua AA, Weiss ST, Gold DR. Day care attendance in

the first year of life and illnesses of the upper and lower respiratory tract in children with a familial history of atopy. Pediatrics. sept 1999;104(3 Pt 1):495- 500.

31. Nystad W, Skrondal A, Magnus P. Day care attendance, recurrent respiratory tract infections and asthma. Int J Epidemiol. oct 1999;28(5):882- 887.

32. Nafstad P, Hagen JA, Oie L, Magnus P, Jaakkola JJ. Day care centers and respiratory health. Pediatrics. avr 1999;103(4 Pt 1):753- 758.

33. Strangert K. Respiratory illness in preschool children with different forms of day care. Pediatrics. févr 1976;57(2):191- 196.

34. Hurwitz ES, Gunn WJ, Pinsky PF, Schonberger LB. Risk of respiratory illness associated with day-care attendance: a nationwide study. Pediatrics. janv 1991;87(1):62- 69.

35. McCutcheon H, Woodward A. Acute respiratory illness in the first year of primary school related to previous attendance at child care. Aust N Z J Public Health. févr 1996;20(1):49- 53.

36. Ministère de la santé. Plan national d'alerte sur les antibiotiques, 2011- 2016 [Internet]. 2011. Disponible sur: http://www.sante.gouv.fr/IMG/pdf/plan_antibiotiques_2011- 2016_DEFINITIF.pdf

37. Agence du médicament. Etude de la prescription et de la consommation des antibiotiques en ambulatoire. 1998.

38. Mémo Infections respiratoires hautes: Antibiothérapie chez l'enfant après avis de la HAS conformément aux avis de la transparence sur les différents produits. Assurance Maladie; 2012.

39. Mémo Rhinopharyngite: Chez l'enfant et l'adulte D'après les recommandations de l'AFSSAPS (octobre 2005) en collaboration avec la HAS. Assurance Maladie; 2009.

40. BELLON G, GRIMPREL E, CHEVALIER B. Conférnce de consensus: Prise en charge de la bronchiolite du nourrisson. Agence Nationale d'Acreditation et d'Évaluation en Santé; Union Régionale des Médecins Libéraux; 2000.

41. PORTIER H, CHOUTET P, CREMIEUX A-C, TRÉMOLIÈRES F, COHEN R. Bronchite aigue de l'adulte sain et de l'enfant. Assurance Maladie;

42. Mémo Otite moyenne aiguë: chez l'enfant de plus de trois mois d'après les recommandations de l'AFSSAPS (octobre 2005) en collaboration avec la HAS. Assurance Maladie; 2009.

43. Mémo Sinusite Prise en charge de la sinusite aiguë de l'adulte d'après les recommandations de l'AFSSAPS (octobre 2005) en collaboration avec la HAS. Assurance Maladie; 2009.

44. Infections ORL et bronchiques des jeunes enfants: Guide à l'usage des professionnelsen charge de l'accueil des jeunes enfants. AFSSAPS; 2006.

45. Résistances bactériennes en France :focus sur les dernières données.

Assurance Maladie; 2010.

46. Alho OP, Läärä E, Oja H. What is the natural history of recurrent acute otitis media in infancy? J Fam Pract. sept 1996;43(3):258- 264.

47. Société Française de Médecine Générale. Observatoire de Médecine Générale [Internet]. 2010. Disponible sur: http://omg.sfmg.org
48. PEPIN S, RICORDEAU P. La consommation d'antibiotiques : situation en France au regard des autres pays européens. Point Repère [Internet]. nov 2006;(6).

49. ANSM. Dix ans d'évolution des consommations d'antibiotiques en France [Internet]. 2012.

XI. ANNEXES :

A. ANNEXE N°1 : L'OBSERVATOIRE DE MEDECINE GENERALE :

1. Objectifs de l'Observatoire de la MG :

Les informations produites par l'OMG, proche de la réalité de la pratique et des contraintes de la médecine générale, alimentent des travaux de recherche réalisés par la SFMG au niveau national mais aussi des projets de recherches internationaux. L'OMG contribue ainsi à faire progresser la connaissance des pathologies, l'efficacité de la prise en charge et l'évolution de la pratique en médecine générale. Il permet notamment d'éclairer la formation médicale initiale et continue et d'étayer l'élaboration de référentiels professionnels.

L'OMG produit régulièrement des données sur l'activité des médecins généralistes et permet à ces derniers de comparer leurs pratiques à la pratique générale et de repositionner leur stratégie décisionnelle de façon constructive.

2. Définition du résultat de consultation :

Le résultat de consultation (RC) est l'ensemble des conclusions diagnostiques du médecin au terme de la séance, pondérées par une position diagnostique et un code suivi.

Le terme de « Résultat de Consultation » est utilisé pour décrire le contenu de la consultation, à savoir, soit un symptôme, soit un syndrome, soit un tableau de maladie ou un diagnostic certifié.

De nombreux médecins utilisent le Dictionnaire des Résultats de Consultation pour documenter leurs dossiers médicaux et structurer la réflexion sur leurs prises de décision. Ils appréhendent ainsi plus facilement les problèmes pris en charge, leur niveau de risque et l'étendue de leur espace de liberté.

3. Dictionnaire des Résultats de Consultation :

Le Dictionnaire des Résultats de Consultation (DRC) est un recueil des RC classés par ordre alphabétique. Il contient à la fois 271 RC et 18 dénominations hors listes. Le DRC n'est pas une classification mais une nomenclature d'« ensemble des termes techniques d'une science » classés par ordre alphabétique, un outil conçu par la SFMG à partir des concepts novateurs du Dr Robert N. Braun.

Le DRC permet de saisir son dossier médical avec un haut niveau de certitude: en effet chaque définition comprend des critères dont certains sont obligatoires.

La notion de "Position Diagnostique" et de "Diagnostic Etiologique Critique" permet au praticien de gérer l'incertitude diagnostique en s'appuyant sur une certitude clinique. Cette préoccupation est fondamentale, en particulier devant un cas non caractéristique. Le DRC est un moyen d'entrer dans une démarche de "gestion du risque".

Le DRC permet aussi le recueil de données.

Le DRC est un langage commun. Il permet donc une analyse des pratiques. Les données recueillies lors de la saisie des Résultats de Consultation sont stockées dans une base de données et mises en ligne sur l'Observatoire de la Médecine Générale. Dans les 10 millions de résultats de consultation, 71 % sont des symptômes isolés ou des syndromes - 29 % des tableaux de maladie ou des diagnostics certifiés.

4. Correspondance CIM 10 :

Il y a un encodage des Résultats de Consultation avec la Classification

Internationale des Maladies (CIM10) : cela permet une analyse des pratiques à l'échelle internationale

B. ANNEXE N°2 : RESULTATS DE CONSULTATION :

RC	Total	% de RC	% Cumulé
EXAMEN SYSTEMATIQUE ET PREVENTION	6977	14%	14%
VACCINATION	3743	8%	22%
ETAT FEBRILE	**6039**	**13%**	**35%**
RHINOPHARYNGITE - RHUME	**5136**	**11%**	**45%**
ASTHME	874	2%	47%
OTITE MOYENNE	**2738**	**6%**	**53%**
ETAT MORBIDE AFEBRILE	**3327**	**7%**	**60%**
TOUX	**1228**	**3%**	**62%**
BRONCHITE AIGUË	**1283**	**3%**	**65%**
ECZEMA	628	1%	66%
REACTION TUBERCULINIQUE	657	1%	68%
RHINITE	**489**	**1%**	**69%**
ANGINE (AMYGDALITE - PHARYNGITE)	**1947**	**4%**	**73%**
REFLUX-PYROSIS-OESOPHAGITE	177	0%	73%
PLAINTE ABDOMINALE	595	1%	74%
OBESITE	113	0%	75%
CONJONCTIVITE	675	1%	76%
DERMATOSE	700	1%	77%
DIARRHEE (ISOLEE, NON INFECTIEUSE)	**422**	**1%**	**78%**
CONSTIPATION	274	1%	79%
PREPUCE ADHERENCE-PHIMOSIS	191	0%	79%
DIARRHEE NAUSEE VOMISSEMENT	**848**	**2%**	**81%**
PSYCHIQUE (TROUBLE)	85	0%	81%
CERUMEN (BOUCHON DE)	333	1%	82%
SOUFFLE CARDIAQUE	147	0%	82%
DENOMINATION HORS-LISTE	173	0%	83%
ENURESIE PSYCHOGENE	128	0%	83%
ANOMALIE POSTURALE	160	0%	83%
PIED (ANOMALIE STATIQUE)	148	0%	83%
SUITE OPERATOIRE	198	0%	84%
VERRUE	229	0%	84%

LANGAGE ORAL ET ECRIT (TROUBLE DU)	125	0%	85%
VARICELLE	451	1%	85%
DHL 06 - Maladie du système nerveux	52	0%	86%
MOLLUSCUM CONTAGIOSUM	135	0%	86%
PNEUMOPATHIE AIGUE	103	0%	86%
DEPRESSION	44	0%	86%
INSOMNIE	117	0%	86%
PROCEDURE ADMINISTRATIVE	135	0%	87%
URTICAIRE	211	0%	87%
SURCHARGE PONDERALE	76	0%	87%
NAUSEE OU VOMISSEMENT	343	1%	88%
ENTORSE	130	0%	88%
ARTHROPATHIE-PERIARTHROPATHIE	123	0%	89%
DHL 18 - Symptômes, signes et résultats anormaux, non classés ailleurs	90	0%	89%
CONTUSION	280	1%	89%
ERYTHEME FESSIER NOURRISSON	146	0%	90%
IMPETIGO	185	0%	90%
DIFFICULTE SCOLAIRE	83	0%	90%
FRACTURE	46	0%	90%
ANXIETE - ANGOISSE	67	0%	90%
CYSTITE - CYSTALGIE	124	0%	91%
OTITE EXTERNE	120	0%	91%
PLAIE	165	0%	91%
PANARIS	76	0%	91%
ECZEMA FACE NOURRISSON	62	0%	92%
DHL 05 - Troubles mentaux et du comportement	28	0%	92%
DERMITE SEBORRHEIQUE	46	0%	92%
STOMATITE - GLOSSITE	137	0%	92%
CEPHALEE	123	0%	92%
ANEMIE FERRIPRIVE - CARENCE EN FER	63	0%	92%
SINUSITE	56	0%	92%
NAEVUS	46	0%	93%
PIQURE D'INSECTE	172	0%	93%
VULVITE-VAGINITE	108	0%	93%
NERVOSISME	44	0%	93%

DHL 14 - Maladies de l'appareil génito-urinaire	39	0%	93%
DOULEUR NON CARACTERISTIQUE	188	0%	94%
OTALGIE	149	0%	94%
ADENOPATHIE	101	0%	94%
ONGLE (PATHOLOGIE DE)	62	0%	94%
REACTION A SITUATION EPROUVANTE	57	0%	94%
ASTHENIE - FATIGUE	69	0%	95%
TARSALGIE - METATARSALGIE	52	0%	95%
DHL 17 - Malformations congénitales et anomalies chromosomiques	17	0%	95%
TUMEFACTION	81	0%	95%
BLESSURES COMBINEES LEGERES	70	0%	95%
BALANO-POSTHITE	79	0%	95%
AMAIGRISSEMENT	30	0%	95%
ECZEMA PALMO-PLANTAIRE DYSHIDROSIQUE	30	0%	95%
DHL 13 - Maladie du syst ostéo-articulaire, des muscles et du tissu conjonctif	26	0%	95%
BACTERIURIE - PYURIE	30	0%	95%
HYPOTHYROIDIE	12	0%	95%
INTERTRIGO	76	0%	96%
HERNIE - EVENTRATION	29	0%	96%
CONTRACEPTION	10	0%	96%
PRURIT LOCALISE	70	0%	96%
DHL 01 - Certaines maladies infectieuses et parasitaires	60	0%	96%
ABCES SUPERFICIEL	56	0%	96%
BRULURE	41	0%	96%
VERTIGE - ETAT VERTIGINEUX	21	0%	96%
EPISTAXIS	61	0%	96%
ENROUEMENT	51	0%	96%
LOMBALGIE	35	0%	97%
COMPORTEMENT (TROUBLES)	28	0%	97%
INCONTINENCE URINAIRE	18	0%	97%
MIGRAINE	18	0%	97%
HYPERLIPIDÉMIE	9	0%	97%
ANOMALIE BIOLOGIQUE SANGUINE	45	0%	97%
PRURIT GENERALISE	17	0%	97%
ANOREXIE - BOULIMIE	11	0%	97%

MAL DE GORGE	63	0%	97%
PARASITOSE DIGESTIVE	51	0%	97%
DENT	46	0%	97%
DYSPNEE	46	0%	97%
TENOSYNOVITE	40	0%	97%
ACCES ET CRISE	31	0%	97%
DHL 07 - Maladies de l'œil et de ses annexes	25	0%	97%
COLIQUE (SYNDROME)	24	0%	98%
CHALAZION	22	0%	98%
CHEVEUX (CHUTE)	19	0%	98%
CONVULSION FEBRILE	13	0%	98%
DHL 08 - Mal de l'oreille et de l'apophyse mastoïde	13	0%	98%
PYELONEPHRITE AIGUE	10	0%	98%
DHL 03 - Mal du sang, des organes hémato. et certaines du syst. Immunitaire	7	0%	98%
GLAUCOME	7	0%	98%
CERVICALGIE	55	0%	98%
SURDITE	41	0%	98%
ABDOMEN DOULOUREUX AIGU	27	0%	98%
FURONCLE - ANTHRAX	20	0%	98%
GALE	16	0%	98%
LUXATION	9	0%	98%
EPILEPSIE	7	0%	98%
ANEMIE (NON FERRIPRIVE)	6	0%	98%
APHTE	57	0%	98%
HERPES	34	0%	98%
POLLAKIURIE	28	0%	98%
MALAISE - EVANInf.SSEMENT	27	0%	98%
DOULEUR PELVIENNE	21	0%	98%
TIC	20	0%	98%
APPETIT (PERTE D')	14	0%	99%
TROUBLE DU RYTHME (AUTRE)	10	0%	99%
BRONCHITE CHRONIQUE	7	0%	99%
MENORRAGIE-METRORRAGIE	6	0%	99%
DHL 09 - Maladie de l'appareil circulatoire	4	0%	99%
FOLLICULITE SUPERFICIELLE	32	0%	99%

ŒIL (TROUBLE DE LA VISION)	29	0%	99%
DHL 12 - Maladie de la peau et des tissus cellulaires sous cutané	27	0%	99%
ACNE	25	0%	99%
DORSALGIE	25	0%	99%
PIED D'ATHLETE	24	0%	99%
MORSURE - GRIFFURE	22	0%	99%
LUCITE - ALLERGIE SOLAIRE	21	0%	99%
EPIGASTRALGIE	11	0%	99%
DHL 10 - Maladies de l'appareil respiratoire	10	0%	99%
URETRITE	9	0%	99%
PITYRIASIS ROSE DE GIBERT	8	0%	99%
PROBLEME FAMILIAL	8	0%	99%
CICATRICE	7	0%	99%
PSORIASIS	7	0%	99%
TABAGISME	5	0%	99%
DHL - Autres	4	0%	99%
DHL 16 - Certaines affections dont origine période périnatale	4	0%	99%
HUMEUR DEPRESSIVE	4	0%	99%
GOITRE	3	0%	99%
TRAUMATISME CRANIOCEREBRAL	26	0%	99%
OEIL (TRAUMATISME)	17	0%	99%
ZONA	17	0%	99%
GINGIVITE	15	0%	99%
MYALGIE	15	0%	99%
DHL 11 - Maladies de l'appareil digestif	13	0%	99%
OEDEME DE QUINCKE - URTICAIRE GEANTE	11	0%	99%
DYSURIE	9	0%	99%
HEMATURIE	9	0%	99%
METEORISME	8	0%	99%
IATROGENE - EFFET INDESIRABLE D'UNE THERAPEUTIQUE	7	0%	99%
TYMPAN (PERFORATION TRAUMATIQUE)	5	0%	99%
ECZEMA PALMO-PLANTAIRE FISSURAIRE	4	0%	99%
ORCHI-EPIDIDYMITE	4	0%	99%
FISSURE ANALE	25	0%	100%
ECCHYMOSE SPONTANEE	21	0%	100%

RECTORRAGIES	13	0%	100%
ORGELET	11	0%	100%
SEIN (TUMEFACTION)	11	0%	100%
CORPS ETRANGER DANS CAVITE NATURELLE	10	0%	100%
MOLLUSCUM PENDULUM	9	0%	100%
KYSTE SYNOVIAL	7	0%	100%
OEIL (LARMOIEMENT)	7	0%	100%
PHOBIE	6	0%	100%
ACOUPHENE	5	0%	100%
EPAULE (TENOSYNOVITE)	4	0%	100%
CRAMPE MUSCULAIRE	3	0%	100%
ERYSIPELE	2	0%	100%
ACCIDENT VASCULAIRE CEREBRAL	1	0%	100%
HYPERURICEMIE	1	0%	100%
OEDEME LOCALISE	11	0%	100%
PITYRIASIS VERSICOLOR	11	0%	100%
CORPS ETRANGER SOUS-CUTANE	10	0%	100%
KYSTE SEBACE	8	0%	100%
FECALOME	7	0%	100%
PRECORDIALGIE	7	0%	100%
SEIN (AUTRE)	6	0%	100%
MUSCLE (ELONGATION-DECHIRURE)	5	0%	100%
COR - DURILLON	4	0%	100%
HEMORROIDE	4	0%	100%
LYMPHANGITE	3	0%	100%
PLAINTES POLYMORPHES (TROUBLES SOMATOFORMES)	3	0%	100%
ALBUMINURIE	2	0%	100%
BLESSURES COMBINEES SEVERES	2	0%	100%
COCCYDYNIE	2	0%	100%
COLIQUE NEPHRETIQUE	2	0%	100%
DHL 04 - Maladies endocriniennes, nutritionnelle et métaboliques	2	0%	100%
ENGELURE	2	0%	100%
LEUCORRHEE	2	0%	100%
LITHIASE URINAIRE	2	0%	100%
NEVRALGIE - NEVRITE	2	0%	100%

ARTHROSE	1	0%	100%
DIABETE DE TYPE 1	1	0%	100%
DYSMENORRHEE	1	0%	100%
EPICONDYLITE	1	0%	100%
HALLUX VALGUS	1	0%	100%
HEMORRAGIE SOUS-CONJONCTIVALE	1	0%	100%
HYPOTENSION ORTHOSTATIQUE	1	0%	100%
MYCOSE UNGUEALE	1	0%	100%
PALPITATION-ERETHISME CARDIAQUE	1	0%	100%
PARESTHESIE DES MEMBRES	1	0%	100%
SYNDROME DE RAYNAUD	1	0%	100%
SYNDROME PREMENSTRUEL	1	0%	100%
TACHYCARDIE PAROXYSTIQUE	1	0%	100%
TREMBLEMENT	1	0%	100%
ULCERE DE JAMBE	1	0%	100%

C. ANNEXE N°3 : DEFINITIONS DES DIX PATHOLOGIES INFECTIEUSES SELECTIONNEES SELON LE DICTIONNAIRE DES RESULTATS DE CONSULTATION :

Observatoire de la Médecine Générale 2010 – SFMG

++++   Signifie que **le critère est obligatoire** pour retenir cette définition
++ X | Signifie le **choix d'au moins X critères** dans la liste
+ -   Signifie **avec ou sans** ce critère. Il s'agit de compléments sémiologiques facultatifs

1. ANGINE (AMYGDALITE - PHARYNGITE)

Critères
++++ ROUGEUR DE L'OROPHARYNX
  ++1| diffuse du pharynx
  ++1| d'une (ou des) amygdale(s)
++++ ABSENCE D'ÉCOULEMENT NASAL CARACTÉRISTIQUE

+ - douleur
+ - fièvre ou sensation de fièvre
+ - hypertrophie
+ - enduit pultacé
+ - adénopathie sous angulo-maxillaire
+ - unilatérale

+ - vésicules
+ - ulcération
+ - fausses membranes

+ - toux
+ - vomissement
+ - douleur abdominale

+ - score de Mac Isaac >= 4
+ - TDR positif
+ - présence bactérienne

+ - récidive

asymptomatique

2. BRONCHITE AIGUË

Critères
++++ TOUX
++++ RÂLES RONFLANTS DIFFUS MODIFIÉS PAR LA TOUX
++++ ABSENCE DE BRONCHITE CHRONIQUE (BRONCHITE CHRONIQUE = TOUX+
    EXPECTORATION AU MOINS 3 MOIS PAR AN DEPUIS 2 ANS)

+ - râles sibilants (surtout au début de l'épisode)
+ - dyspnée
+ - expectoration
+ - fièvre ou sensation de fièvre

+ - récidive

asymptomatique

3. DIARRHEE NAUSEE VOMISSEMENT

Critères
++++ SELLES FRÉQUENTES, MOLLES OU LIQUIDES

++1| NAUSÉES
++1| VOMISSEMENTS

+ - borborygme
+ - cas semblables dans l'entourage
+ - perte de poids
+ - abattement, lassitude, myalgies, céphalées, courbatures
+ - douleur abdominale
+ - déshydratation
+ - glaires
+ - sang dans les selles
+ - fièvre ou sensation de fièvre
+ - retour de voyage

+ - récidive

asymptomatique

4. ÉTAT MORBIDE AFÉBRILE

Critères
++++ ASSOCIATION DE SYMPTÔMES ET SIGNES GÉNÉRAUX ET LOCAUX
++++ NON CARACTÉRISTIQUE ET NON CLASSABLE AILLEURS
++++ ABSENCE DE FIÈVRE OU SENSATION DE FIÈVRE

+ - abattement, lassitude, inappétence (incapacité au travail, frissons, " enfant grognon ")
+ - céphalée
+ - état vertigineux
+ - courbatures, myalgies
+ - obstruction, écoulement nasal
+ - douleurs sinusiennes spontanées ou provoquées
+ - symptôme ou signe pharyngé ou amygdalien
+ - modification de la voix
+ - toux
+ - expectoration minime, non caractéristique
+ - signes auscultatoires pulmonaires non significatifs
+ - sensation de brûlure rétrosternale
+ - auriculaire : otalgie, tympans un peu rouges ou discrètement modifiés
+ - oculaire : larmoiement, rougeur conjonctivale
+ - nausées
+ - vomissements
+ - douleur abdominale
+ - selles molles, diarrhée
+ - pollakiurie
+ - brûlures mictionnelles
+ - exanthème
+ - adénopathies
+ - après vaccination

+ - récidive

asymptomatique

5. ÉTAT FÉBRILE

Critères
++++ FIÈVRE OU SENSATION DE FIÈVRE
++1| isolée
+ - frissons, sueurs, courbatures
++1| associée à des symptômes et signes généraux et locaux
++++ NON CARACTÉRISTIQUE ET NON CLASSABLE AILLEURS
+ - abattement, lassitude, inappétence (incapacité au travail, frissons, " enfant grognon ")
+ - céphalée
+ - état vertigineux
+ - courbatures, myalgies
+ - obstruction, écoulement nasal
+ - douleurs sinusiennes spontanées ou provoquées
+ - symptôme ou signe pharyngé ou amygdalien
+ - modification de la voix
+ - toux
+ - expectoration minime, non caractéristique
+ - signes auscultatoires pulmonaires non significatifs
+ - sensation de brûlure rétrosternale
+ - auriculaire : otalgie, tympans un peu rouges ou discrètement modifiés
+ - oculaire : larmoiement, rougeur conjonctivale
+ - nausées
+ - vomissements
+ - douleur abdominale
+ - douleur lombaire uni ou bilatérale
+ - selles molles, diarrhée
+ - pollakiurie
+ - brûlures mictionnelles
+ - urines troubles
+ - exanthème
+ - adénopathies
+ - récidive
asymptomatique

6. OTITE MOYENNE

Critères
++++ TYMPAN(S) MODIFIÉ(S)
  ++1| rouge vif
  ++1| rosé ou ambré
  ++1| mat ou blanchâtre
  ++1| bombé (partiellement ou totalement)
  ++1| rétracté
  ++1| phlycténulaire ou phlycténulo-hémorragique
  ++1| épaissi
  ++1| niveaux liquides (ou bulles hydroaériques)
  ++1| perforation spontanée ou après paracentèse (exclus les traumatismes récents)
  ++1| autre (à préciser en commentaire)

+ - droite
+ - gauche

+ - fièvre ou sensation de fièvre
+ - otalgie
+ - otorrhée ou otorragie
+ - hypoacousie
+ - résultat d'impédancemétrie

+ - récidive

asymptomatique

7. PNEUMOPATHIE AIGUE

Critères
++1| SIGNES CLINIQUES
   ++++ fièvre ou frissons
   ++++ râles crépitants en foyer
   ++++ toux
   ++++ douleur thoracique localisée

++1| SIGNES RADIOLOGIQUES FOCALISÉS AVEC IMAGES PARENCHYMATEUSES
      DE DISTRIBUTION PLUS OU MOINS SEGMENTAIRE OU LOBAIRE
   ++1| fièvre
   ++1| toux
   ++1| douleur thoracique localisée
   ++1| râles crépitants en foyer

+ - expectoration
+ - dyspnée avec battements des ailes du nez du nourrisson
+ - douleur abdominale
+ - état général altéré
+ - submatité
+ - souffle tubaire
+ - augmentation des vibrations vocales
+ - germe

+ - récidive

Asymptomatique

8. RHINOPHARYNGITE - RHUME

Critères
++1| RHINORRHÉE ANTÉRIEURE OU POSTÉRIEURE
   ++1| claire
   ++1| muco-purulente
++1| OBSTRUCTION NASALE

++++ D'APPARITION RÉCENTE (DE QUELQUES HEURES À QUELQUES JOURS)
++++ SANS SIGNES GÉNÉRAUX MARQUÉS

+ - fièvre
+ - toux
+ - gêne à la déglutition
+ - sécrétion oculaire purulente
+ - rougeur pharyngée
+ - adénopathie sous angulo-maxillaire

+ - récidive

asymptomatique

9. SINUSITE

Critères
++1| DOULEUR
    ++1| sinus frontaux
    ++1| sinus maxillaire droit
    ++1| sinus maxillaire gauche

   ++++ spontanée
   ++++ retrouvée à la palpation
   ++++ écoulement nasal purulent
    ++1| antérieur
    ++1| postérieur

+ - lancinante
+ - majorée par mouvements tête
+ - provoquée percussion dentaire supérieure
+ - toux
+ - fièvre ou sensation de fièvre
+ - opacité/flou à la transillumination
+ - non-réponse aux vaso-constricteurs locaux

++1| SIGNES D'IMAGERIE (À LA RADIOGRAPHIE OU AU SCANNER)

++1| PUS À LA PONCTION DES SINUS

+ - récidive
asymptomatique

10. TOUX

Critères
++++ TOUX
++++ SANS SYMPTÔME OU SIGNE ÉVOQUANT UN AUTRE RC
+ - toux rapportée
+ - grasse
+ - sèche
+ - rauque
+ - quinteuse
+ - d'effort
+ - émétisante
+ - diurne
+ - au décubitus
+ - au procubitus
+ - récidive
asymptomatique

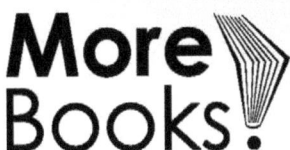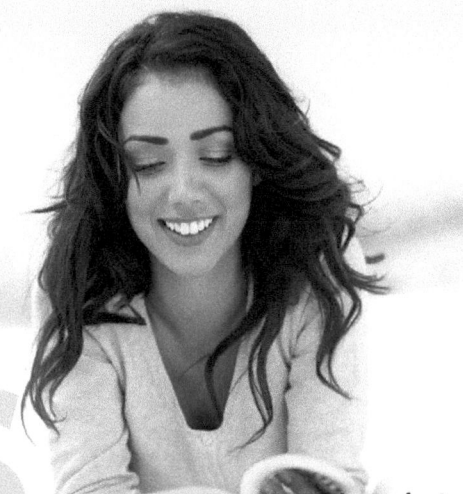

I want morebooks!

Buy your books fast and straightforward online - at one of the world's fastest growing online book stores! Environmentally sound due to Print-on-Demand technologies.

Buy your books online at
www.get-morebooks.com

Achetez vos livres en ligne, vite et bien, sur l'une des librairies en ligne les plus performantes au monde!
En protégeant nos ressources et notre environnement grâce à l'impression à la demande.

La librairie en ligne pour acheter plus vite
www.morebooks.fr

OmniScriptum Marketing DEU GmbH
Heinrich-Böcking-Str. 6-8
D - 66121 Saarbrücken
Telefax: +49 681 93 81 567-9

info@omniscriptum.com
www.omniscriptum.com

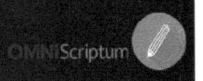

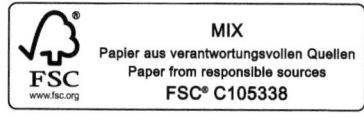

Printed by Books on Demand GmbH, Norderstedt / Germany

Zhiqiang Zhang

Finance – Fundamental Problems and Solutions

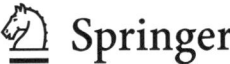 Springer

Zhiqiang Zhang
Business School
Renmin University of China
Beijing
People's Republic of China

ISSN 2191-5482
ISSN 2191-5490 (electronic)
ISBN 978-3-642-30511-5
ISBN 978-3-642-30512-2 (eBook)
DOI 10.1007/978-3-642-30512-2
Springer Heidelberg New York Dordrecht London

Library of Congress Control Number: 2013936521

© The Author(s) 2013

This work is subject to copyright. All rights are reserved by the Publisher, whether the whole or part of the material is concerned, specifically the rights of translation, reprinting, reuse of illustrations, recitation, broadcasting, reproduction on microfilms or in any other physical way, and transmission or information storage and retrieval, electronic adaptation, computer software, or by similar or dissimilar methodology now known or hereafter developed. Exempted from this legal reservation are brief excerpts in connection with reviews or scholarly analysis or material supplied specifically for the purpose of being entered and executed on a computer system, for exclusive use by the purchaser of the work. Duplication of this publication or parts thereof is permitted only under the provisions of the Copyright Law of the Publisher's location, in its current version, and permission for use must always be obtained from Springer. Permissions for use may be obtained through RightsLink at the Copyright Clearance Center. Violations are liable to prosecution under the respective Copyright Law.

The use of general descriptive names, registered names, trademarks, service marks, etc. in this publication does not imply, even in the absence of a specific statement, that such names are exempt from the relevant protective laws and regulations and therefore free for general use.

While the advice and information in this book are believed to be true and accurate at the date of publication, neither the authors nor the editors nor the publisher can accept any legal responsibility for any errors or omissions that may be made. The publisher makes no warranty, express or implied, with respect to the material contained herein.

Printed on acid-free paper

Springer is part of Springer Science+Business Media (www.springer.com)

Preface

Finance as an independent science has been exiting for 60 years (Since Harry Markowitz published his Portfolio theory paper in 1952). However, many of the fundamental problems in finance remain unsolved, such as how to value a stock, how to determine the optimal capital structure of a firm, how to determine an appropriate discount rate accounting for total risk of an investment rather than only systematic risk as in Sharpe's capital asset pricing model (1964), etc.

Financial practice has been calling for the solutions to these fundamental problems.In absence of the basic solutions to these problems, more and more practical problems have been cumulated, such as what is the fair P/E (price–earnings ratio) of a stock or a market, what is the appropriate method to measure the bubble of a stock or a market, what is the right approach to calculate a firm's bankruptcy cost arising from debt financing, what is the efficient way to determine the optimal capital structure of a firm, why does "financial conservatism" spread so extensively and persistently, what is the quantitative relationship between total risk and return, how can we determine a (total) risk-adjusted discount rate for valuing an asset or evaluating a project, etc. In shortage of efficient and reliable theoretical solutions, financial practitioners have to make their investment and financing decisions relying only on their intuitions or industrial conventions.

This book records my efforts and solutions to these fundamental problems. Chapter 1 explores the fundamental features of finance, which is necessary for efficiently understanding and solving financial problems. Chapter 2 discusses a financial paradox (growth paradox), which is helpful for examining our financial reasoning and identifying the current phrase of financial theory. Chapter 3 develops a brand new valuation method—valuation based on required payback period, which can overcome most of the limitations of discounted cash flow method (DCF, such as Gordon growth model) and hence is more powerful in stock valuation. Chapter 4 develops a series of brand new models for incorporating total risk into valuation, which include a risk equivalent (coefficient) model, a certainty equivalent (coefficient) model, a risk premium model, and a new CAPM. Chapter 5 develops a series of brand new models for valuing tax shield and bankruptcy cost as well as for determining the optimal capital structure, hence solves the problem of optimal capital structure and gets more convincing explanations for various capital structure puzzles.

The above fundamental problems as well as the relevant financial concepts and models, such as P/E ratio, Gordon model, CAPM, certainty equivalent, tax shield, bankruptcy cost, optimal leverage, etc., absorb me day and night. My solutions may not be perfect, but they are surely simple and innovative method with theoretical soundness. Since there are no reliable solutions to these fundamental problems in prevailing finance books and journals, the solutions in this book can surely benefit students, researchers, analysts, and practitioners as irreplaceable solutions and supplement theories to prevailing financial theories before the better solutions and theories are emerged.

The solutions in this book have vast application potential mainly in valuation, investment, capital budgeting, risk management, financing, and capital structure decision, etc. Specially speaking, investment banks can use the brand new valuation method and stock valuation model in their operations of IPO, P&A; hedge fund and other investment institutions can use the new stock valuation model and the new theoretical ratio models in their investment selections and decisions. Most business firms can use the new CAPM to improve their capital budgeting and project investment decisions; and use the optimal capital structure model to improve their financing decisions. Commercial banks, rating agencies, and insurance companies can use the certainty equivalent model and optimal capital structure model to evaluate the risk of their customers and make better judgments and decisions.

The author thanks all the academic and practical experts, including K. Thomas Liaw, Ronnie Qi, Gerry John, Jiansheng Liu, Ruqi Wang, Yaping Yin, Chang Song, Mingxuan Yu, Dongming Liu, Dongping Qi, Jiwen Song, Shufang Xiao, Wuxiang Zhu, Zhengwei Wang, Jun Zhu, Shaohao Wang, Qiang Zhao, Jin Cui, etc., for their various helps and insightful comments during my research and writing. Thanks to Mr. Toby Chai and other employees in Springer for their enthusiastic help and efforts for publishing this book.

I have been extremely busy year after year for seeking all the solutions in this book and have spared little time to perform my duties in my family. Thanks to my father, my mother, thanks for their consistent support from beginning to end; thanks to my wife and my son, they has to deal with all troubles I left to them, and endure various hardships because my research cannot obtain any financial support in current research environment.

Finally, thanks to all people who are kind-hearted to the development of financial theory, since there has been seldom breakthrough discovery in financial theory for recent 30 years though the financial research has been booming strongly.

All the faults and errors in the book are my own. Your criticisms and comments on my reasoning and models as well as writing are warmly welcomed.

August 2012   Zhiqiang Zhang

Contents

1 **Finance and its Fundamental Problems** 1
   1.1 Financial Theory and Business Practice. 1
   1.2 Finance in Academic Knowledge Spectrum 3
   1.3 Fundamental Problems in Finance........................... 5
      1.3.1 Financial Decision Criteria. 5
      1.3.2 Fundamental Problems in Finance 6
      1.3.3 Fundamental Problems Remain Unsolved 8

2 **Does a Positive Perpetual Growth Rate Exist?**.................... 9
   2.1 Average Annual Growth Rate Revisit. 9
   2.2 Arithmetic or Geometric Average Growth Rate................ 11
   2.3 ZZ Growth Paradox 12
   2.4 Bankruptcy Probability and Firm Life 14
   2.5 Is Bankruptcy Loss Incorporated into Discount Rate?........... 17
   2.6 The Implied Perpetual Growth Rate.......................... 18
   2.7 The Stage of Finance as a Science 20
   References.. 20

3 **Valuation Based on Required Payback Period** 23
   3.1 Absolute Valuation and Relative Valuation 23
      3.1.1 Absolute Valuation 23
      3.1.2 Relative Evaluation. 24
      3.1.3 Option Pricing Valuation 26
   3.2 Cases When Current Absolute and Relative Valuation Invalid...... 31
   3.3 A New Absolute Valuation Method Based on Required
      Payback Period.. 33
      3.3.1 ZZ Growth Model 34
      3.3.2 Solutions Based on ZZ Growth Model. 35
      3.3.3 Comparison of Gordon model and ZZ Growth Model...... 36
   3.4 The Theoretical Ratio Models 38
      3.4.1 ZZ P/E Model...................................... 38
      3.4.2 ZZ P/B Model...................................... 41
      3.4.3 ZZ P/S Model...................................... 43

		3.5	Some of the Applications of ZZ Growth Model	
			and ZZ Ratio Models	44
		3.5.1	Calculating the Fair-Priced Ratios	44
		3.5.2	Measuring the Market Bubble	46
		3.5.3	Predicting the Change of Stock Price...........	47
	3.6	Summary	50
	References...	50

4 Certainty Equivalent, Risk Premium and Asset Pricing 51
   4.1 Alternatives to Determine a Discount Rate 51
       4.1.1 The Industrial Average Rate of Return.................. 52
       4.1.2 The Opportunity Cost of Capital 52
       4.1.3 The Weighted Average Cost of Capital 53
       4.1.4 The Capital Asset Pricing Model 55
   4.2 Certainty Equivalent and Risk Equivalent 56
       4.2.1 On Certainty Equivalent.............................. 57
       4.2.2 Risk Equivalent Model............................... 58
       4.2.3 Certainty Equivalent Model 61
       4.2.4 Exemplifications..................................... 62
   4.3 Risk Premium and a New CAPM............................ 64
       4.3.1 Modeling Risk Premium and a New CAPM 64
       4.3.2 Comparison Between Sharpe's CAPM and ZZ CAPM..... 65
       4.3.3 Exemplifications..................................... 67
   4.4 Summary 68
   References... 69

5 Tax Shield, Bankruptcy Cost and Optimal Capital Structure 71
   5.1 Firm's Goal and its Capital Structure......................... 71
   5.2 The Potential Benefits and Costs of Debt Financing 72
       5.2.1 General Analyses 72
       5.2.2 MM Model I.. 73
   5.3 Efforts to Value Tax Shield and Bankruptcy Cost 74
       5.3.1 MM Model II 74
       5.3.2 The Trade-Off Model................................ 75
       5.3.3 Other Efforts.. 76
   5.4 Decision-Oriented Valuation of Tax Shield and Bankruptcy Cost... 77
       5.4.1 The Time Horizon 77
       5.4.2 Value the Tax Shield................................ 78
       5.4.3 Value the Bankruptcy Cost........................... 80
   5.5 Decision-Oriented Optimal Capital Structure Model............. 83
       5.5.1 Derivation of the model 83
       5.5.2 Basic Features of the Model.......................... 84
       5.5.3 Basic Insights from the Model........................ 86
       5.5.4 Assumptions of the Model 89

5.6	Some Application Extensions.		90
	5.6.1	Abnormal Growth.	90
	5.6.2	Bankruptcy Expectancy	91
	5.6.3	Market Value Versus Book Value	92
	5.6.4	Guaranteed Debt.	93
	5.6.5	Transaction Costs	94
	5.6.6	Personal Income Tax	95
	5.6.7	Inter-Firm's Investments.	96
5.7	Explanations to Some Capital Structure Puzzles		97
	5.7.1	Why Financial Conservatism	97
	5.7.2	Why No Leverage Target	98
	5.7.3	Why Averse-Change With Profitability	99
	5.7.4	Why Over Stable Leverage.	99
	5.7.5	Why Pecking Order	100
	5.7.6	Why Market Timing	101
	5.7.7	Dynamic Consideration?	102
	5.7.8	Why Not 0 % Debt in Absence of Corporate Tax	102
5.8	Summary		103
Appendix			104
References			107

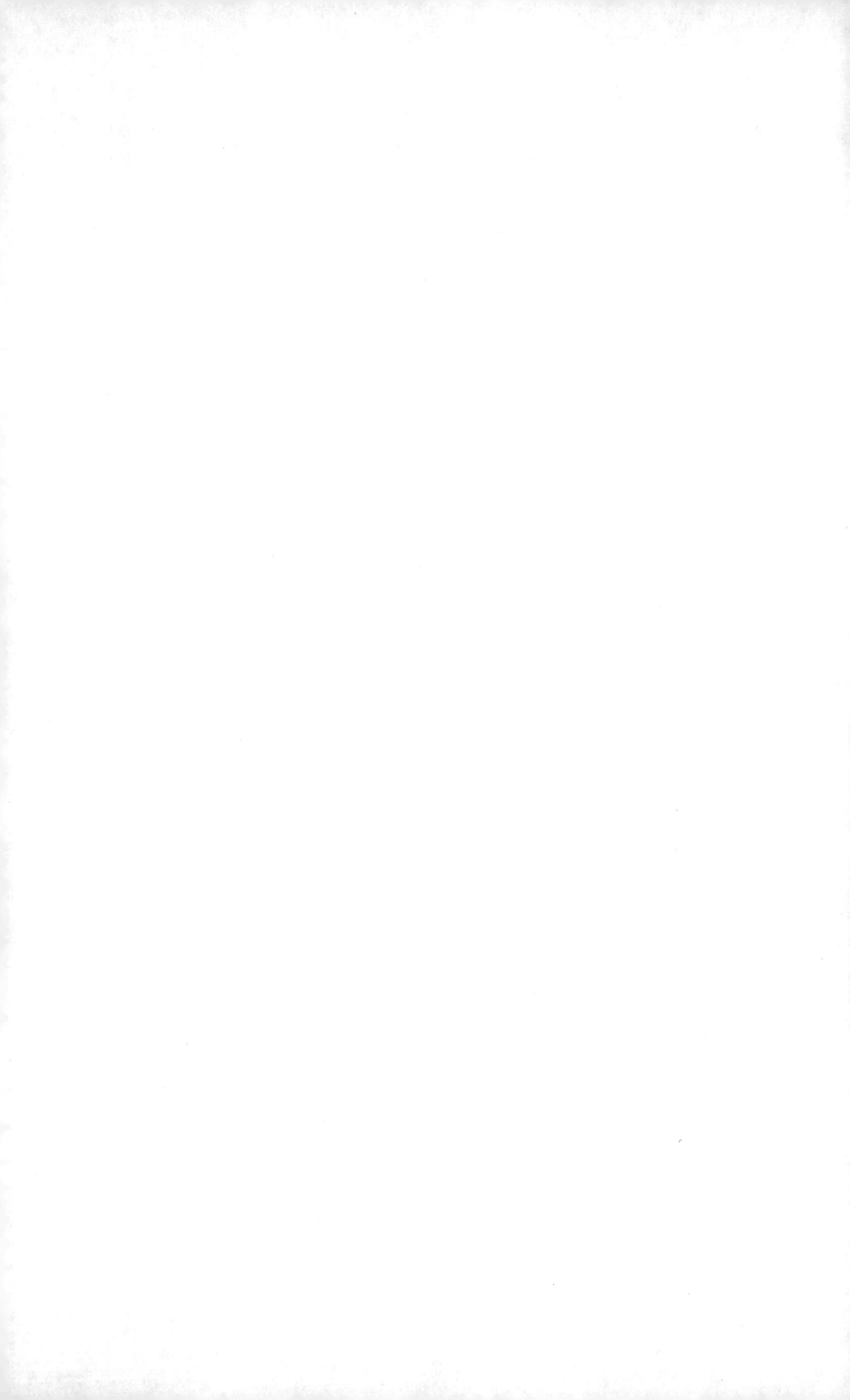

Chapter 1
Finance and its Fundamental Problems

To find efficient solutions to financial problems needs a thorough understanding of finance. There are actually numerous misunderstandings about finance within and beyond the financial community. Those misunderstandings directly damage our judgment on financial research and financial theory, and are some of the reasons why so many fundamental financial problems remain unsolved after 60 years' intensive research.

1.1 Financial Theory and Business Practice

Many people regard financial theory as a tool to make money. This is not very correct. As a social science, financial theory has its unique issues, unique methods as well as unique concepts for us to understand and solve the relevant problems. If we regard financial theory as a tool to make money, our attention may be stopped at actual profit from buying and selling financial assets, regardless the underlying financial principles and problems. That is why we may be confused about some financial problems. Actually, those who are successful in making money are not necessarily successful in theoretical contribution, and vice versa.

Fischer Black (1938–1995) is a good example. Apart from his famous work on option pricing, his works cover numerous financial problems including CAPM and continuous time finance, dividend policy, etc. So many people were struck by the depth of his insight and intuition into economics and finance, even though his manuscripts were rejected often by financial journals. There is a famous story of a presentation by him, to an industry audience, where a smart-aleck kid asked him "if you're so smart, how come you're not rich?" Black replied with a smile "if you're so rich, how come you're not smart?"

Making money is actual the main objective pursued by business rather than that pursued by academy. The academic research should aim at solving theoretical problems. This is by no means that the academic research's interest is totally different from that of the business practice. A theoretical problem should be the common or generalized problem representing a group of practical problems. Solutions of theoretical problems should be useful in practical decision-making. The practitioners may make money by applying a special theoretical solution. However, this is by no means that the inventor of the theoretical solution can also manage to apply the solution to make money, because financial theory is only one of numerous factors in the success to make money. We thus cannot judge a financial theory or model based on how much its inventor makes money.

The importance of practice is over stressed on in most circumstances. Actually, one of the main differences in practice between mankind and animal is just that one is guided by some science or theory, the other is just pure practice. Thus, when we stress on the importance of practice, be careful not to overstate it to the extent that the theory or science is totally unimportant. If we totally abandon science or theory, a foreseeable result is that our society cannot progress anymore; we just repeat the same thing year after year and generation after generation just as what happens in wild animal world. Similarly, if we abandon financial theory or the financial theory is stopped to progress for some reasons, a foreseeable result is that the financial crisis will occur time and time again.

In the range of social affairs, the main function of the social science (such as financial theory) is offering support to the relevant decisions. From a point of view, theory is an answer to a question or a group of questions. We can find answers to various questions. One feature of a good theory is that the question rather than the answer should come from the relevant practice. This is easy to understand. If the question is not from practice, the theory is not guaranteed to be useful even it is a correct answer. But if the answer is also from practice, the theory is definitely useless, because practice itself has solved the problem already, and the theory cannot offer any additional support or help.

A similar argument is that social theory or science should be consistent with reality. This is not very correct either. Theory can be viewed as a statement with premise and conclusion. The main premises of a theory should be consistent with reality; but the conclusion should not be consistent with reality. If a theory, from premises to conclusions, is completely consistent with reality, it must be reality itself, and cannot be a theory anymore. Similarly, such a "theory" is impossible to be useful to guide practical decision-making.

Besides the conclusions, the premises of a theory should not be completely consistent with reality. To obtain a correct conclusion, one premise must not be consistent with reality, which is the irrationality of mankind. The decision-makers may be somehow irrational in reality, which implies that practical decision-making is not necessary to be right exactly. The irrationality is different across persons and times. We can get easily the right answer to the question of "$1 + 1 = ?$". But if the question is "$1 + 1 = ?$ when the calculator is irrational", how can we get a certain or right answer? Obviously, the answer may be any number in such a premise. Similarly, if our premises include the irrationalities of decision-makers, we cannot obtain a correct and certain conclusion, because the irrationalities are fundamentally uncertain in terms of direction and extent. In addition, a rational answer is useful for guiding the practical decision; the irrational answer is usually useless.

We now get some insight. The questions or problems researched in finance should come from practice; but the conclusions or solutions should not be from practice. In practice, decisions must be made within a short time (before deadline); hence the conclusions or solutions may not be correct. However, the theoretical research should pursue the right conclusions or solutions after understanding the question or problem well. Capital structure decision is a good example. Every firm in reality should make its capital structure decision within a given time, regardless whether it really knows how to determine an optimal debt ratio. Therefore, the completion of the practical decision-making does not mean the relevant decision problem is solved; the real solution of a problem is the theoretical one.

1.2 Finance in Academic Knowledge Spectrum

Knowledge is the wealth of mankind. In academic circle, most of the knowledge can be divided into two categories: art and science. Science can be divided further into two categories: natural science and social science. Social science (excluding art) further can be divided into two categories: description science and decision science. Description science try to answer questions like "what is it", "what have been done"; decision science try to answer questions like "what should it be", "what should be done". Examples of description science like history, statistics, accounting, etc. Examples of decision science like economics, finance, management, etc. Those categories of knowledge are shown in Fig. 1.1.

Finance or financial theory belongs to the decision science in social science. It offers concepts, theories and models to help students, researchers, practitioners, etc. understanding financial issues and to support actual financial decision makings. As a decision science, finance is different in many aspects from other kinds of science and knowledge.

Finance as a science is different from art. Arts (in various forms) try to give people sensation or feeling, such as music, painting, novel, film, etc. Finance as a science tries to reveal financial principles and to solve financial problems. A financial research or theory is much different from an art show or exhibition. We can judge the show or exhibition based on our sensation or feeling, but we cannot judge a financial research or theory based on our sensation or feeling before

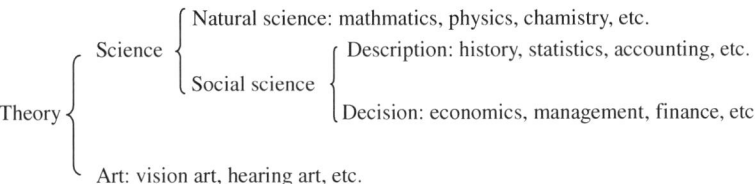

Fig. 1.1 Academic knowledge spectrum

we really understanding the logic or reasoning behind it. It is impossible for an art to be correct or incorrect; but a financial conclusion or theory is possible to be correct or incorrect in most circumstances. The main criteria to judge a financial research or theory should include: whether it is correct in defining and reasoning; how efficient it solves the relevant financial problem; how important and difficult the financial problem is; and how innovative the research method is, etc.

Finance as a social science is different from natural science. To understand some natural phenomenon or issues, scientists sometime resort to data from observations and experiments. This is often an efficient way in natural scientific research, because the conclusion derived from data is certain or reliable. However, the data in social science (hereafter referred to as social data), from observation or experiments, is much different. Social data is the results of people's behavior. The behavior will surely be affected by people's learning effect, mentality, rationality, accidence as well as other complex factors, hence most (if not all) social data is fundamentally uncertain. This implies that it is often impossible to derive a certain or reliable conclusion from social data. Things in financial area are similar. For instance, data of stock price are the result of people's behavior of buying and selling in the market. Numerous factors may change people's buying and selling strategies, such as learning, etc. Therefore, financial theories or solutions should rely mainly on logic-based research rather than data-based research. Actually, even a social data-based conclusion with consistency can hardly be useful, because no one can tell the premises of the based social data. If we do not know the premises of the conclusion, how can we know when and how to use it? Therefore, we should judge a financial solution or theory based on whether its logic or reasoning is correct and rigorous rather than whether it is consistent with some past data.

For instance, to explore the relationship between interest rate and stock price, we can derive a conclusion based on careful reasoning that they are negative related. However, if we observe the actual data, they are negative related in some cases and positive related in other cases. Our conclusion thus depends on the data we collected. The question is: do you really believe the data-based conclusion? If your instant answer is "yes", which conclusion do you really believe, negative related or positive related? Further, when and how will you apply the two contradicted data-based "conclusions"? The embarrassment aroused from these questions reveals that data-based conclusions in finance are very unreliable; and the basic and final judgment should be based on logic or reasoning rather than unstable past data. This is a very important insight for financial studies and reviews.

Finance as a decision science is different from description science. The purpose of description science is to describe what our society like or what people have done. So we can judge the description research or theory based on how it conforms to the reality or practice. However, the purpose of decision science is to improve people's decision. So we definitely cannot judge the conclusion or theory of a decision science based on its consistence with the reality or practice. Rather, the judgment should be based on its improvement of the prevailing decision making. Most of the description sciences aim at describe the past decisions and their consequences, so they can be past data-based research. However, decision making is always future-oriented. Financial decision is not an exception. Therefore, most (if not all) of the financial research should focus on how or what to do based on foreseeable future. This is very important for understanding and solving financial problems.

As a decision science, finance is different from other subjects, such as economics and various management subjects. Comparing to each other, economics is a theoretical science, whereas finance is an applied science. As a theoretical science, economics stresses on principles and does not care much about the feasibility of the theory or model. For instance, many economic models use utility as an independent variable; but utility can hardly be estimated. As an applied science, finance must consider feasibility of the model or theory and should avoid incorporating variable like utility in its model. On the other hand, finance is not a pure applied science; it has some branches as pure applied subjects, such as investment, valuation, risk management, investment and commercial banking, etc. Finance offers theoretical supports rather than techniques in detail to these pure applied subjects.

Further, finance is different from other management or decision subjects. Some management subjects focus on qualitative problems, such as strategy, organization, marketing, etc., whereas finance focuses on quantitative problems. Finance is also different from other quantity-based decision subjects, such as operation management, management science, etc. Finance is a value-based subject with valuation approach as its main and basic technique, whereas other quantity-based subjects are not. Therefore, finance as a science has unique problem, unique method and unique theory. As a unique subject, it is responsible to deal with special and important financial problems.

1.3 Fundamental Problems in Finance

1.3.1 Financial Decision Criteria

Finance as a subject deals with problems in financial practice, including problems mainly in investment and financing (raising fund or capital). Investment is actually buying assets in some forms, such as stocks, bonds as well as substantial assets like real estate, machine, materials, etc. Financing is actually selling assets in some forms, such as issuing stocks, bonds as well as disposing substantial assets. Therefore, to make a good financial decision, it is necessary to know the value of the relevant assets. The ideal case is that the assets sold are proved to be overvalued and the assets bought are proved to be undervalued. Asset value hence is the most important decision criterion in finance.

As value becomes the major criterion of financial decision, asset valuation becomes the theme and basic method of financial theory. Asset value is determined in a more special and clearer way than the value of other general items. This distinguishes finance as an independent subject from other value-based subjects, such as economics. Financial theory thus gains more feasibility for practical application. Economics (especially microeconomics) as more a theoretical subject deals with values and prices of more general items, and cannot take risk and return as value determinants. Economics reveals more general principle of value determination, hence is perceived as the theoretical foundation of finance.

Assets are something opposite to cash. Sales of assets can increase a firm's cash, while purchases of assets will decrease its cash. Assets can be categorized into financial assets and real assets. Financial assets include securities in various forms, some of them are basic securities, such as bank deposits, stocks, bonds; some of them are derivatives, such as futures and options. Real assets include various tangible and intangible assets. The former is something like buildings, machinery, office and operation equipments and inventories of parts or materials, etc. The later is something like goodwill, intellectual property, patents, copyrights, and trademarks, etc. Financial assets are usually more liquid than real assets.

1.3.2 Fundamental Problems in Finance

Asset (financial assets and real assets) value is determined by its future or expected risk and returns (such as earnings and cash flows). Asset value increases as its (expected) returns increase and decreases as its risk increases. These are the basic axioms of asset value determination, and naturally becomes the start point of financial theory and the basic standard to build as well as to judge a financial model.

As an application-oriented subject, finance should offer methods or models to support investment and financing decisions. Investments can be categorized into security (such as stocks, bonds and derivatives in various forms) investment and real asset (such as project) investment. Financing is issuing securities to raise money. Finance thus should offer methods or models to value securities and projects based on the expected returns and risk.

For valuing securities and projects, we need to consider asset future returns. There are multiple ways to measure asset returns. Accounting uses some indicators to record a firm's past returns, such as earnings, net income and cash flows. Asset future returns thus can be forecasted in terms of such measures. In fact, forecast (as a subject) rather than finance is responsible for describing the future cash flows of an asset. Finance as a science is mainly responsible for decision method or model, or how to incorporate the asset returns into its valuation. Forecasted data is the input of financial method or model, and the valuation or decision conclusion is the output of financial method or model.

Risk is uncertainty. In finance, risk is specifically referred to as the uncertainty in asset returns (earnings, cash flows, etc.). The return uncertainty can be measured by the distribution (the extent of decentralization) of the future possible returns. Statistics uses standard deviation (σ) or variance (σ^2) to reflect the distribution of a variable. Risk thus can be measured this way. With a similar reasoning, while it is mainly the responsibility of statistics to offer efficient methods

1.3 Fundamental Problems in Finance

to measure risks; finance as a science is mainly responsible for offering efficient methods to incorporate the risk into asset valuation.

Therefore, given the returns and risk, such as earnings and its variance of an asset, finance should be able to value the asset and support the relevant decision-making. This implies that financial theory has the following basic tasks:

(1) Determining the quantitative relationship between an asset value and its returns, or how the asset returns should being considered in valuation.

(2) Determining the quantitative relationship between an asset value and its risk, or how the asset risk should being considered in valuation.

Absolute valuation and relative valuation are the two traditional valuation methods in finance. Absolute valuation values an asset based on its fundamentals, i.e. its expected risk and return. Relative valuation values an asset based on the prices (or values) of other similar assets (comparables). The philosophy behind absolute valuation is the axiom of "risk and return determine asset value". The philosophy behind relative valuation is a common sense of "similar assets should have similar value".

Currently, absolute valuation is almost equivalent to discounted cash flow method (DCF). According to DCF, value of an asset is the sum of the present value of its future returns (cash flows). Valuing an asset with DCF method, the risk is incorporated into an appropriate discount rate and the returns are incorporated into the future cash flows of the asset. In addition, contingent claim valuation is an advanced valuation method since last seventies, which is specialized in derivatives' valuation, such as options, etc.

Relative valuation is equivalent to ratio method so far, which is mainly used in stock or equity valuation. According to ratio method, value of an asset is close to the product of its value-driver (often earnings, net asset, revenue, etc.) multiplied by a fair ratio (such as Price to earnings ratio or P/E, Price to book value ratio or P/B, Price to sales ratio or P/S). Ratio method obviously depends on the determination of the fair ratios, such as a fair P/E ratio or P/B ratio. The ratio chosen in current relative valuation is around somehow the industrial average or median, which implies that the relative valuation is currently almost a pure practical valuation method and lack of theoretical soundness.

In addition to the asset or security value, for financing decisions, firms have to trade-off between equity capital and debt capital and choose an optimal capital mix. This implies that the problem of optimal capital structure (the ratio of debt in total assets) is also an important problem in financial theory.

In summary, finance as a science thus has to solve the following fundamental problems:

(1) how to consider the future returns of an asset;
(2) how to determine the fair or theoretical ratios of an asset;
(3) how to estimate a discount rate matching the asset risk, or how to consider asset risk in valuation and decision-making;
(4) how to determine the optimal capital structure of a firm.

1.3.3 Fundamental Problems Remain Unsolved

We sort out four fundamental financial problems in last section. Unfortunately, none of these problems is solved in theory so far. As some of the problems are pervasive in finance, such as problem (1), (2) and (3), that one of these problems remain unsolved may be enough to hinder us from solving most of the financial (investment and financing) problems in theory and in practice. For instance, valuation in both stock and project investment as well as stock or bond issuing need to consider the future returns and to estimate a risk-matched discount rate if we depend DCF for valuation.

As DCF method is almost the only theoretical valuation method, if the future returns (given a best forecast) or its risk cannot be correctly considered, the result derived from the DCF will be unreliable. In this case, how can we rely on the financial analyses to make investment and financing decisions? Ratio method is also widely used in practical stock valuation. Since there are so many firms in an industry, the industrial average of the ratio is impossible to be a good estimation of the fair ratio for a special firm. Similarly, there is no reliable method so far to determine an optimal capital structure of a firm. This implies that the decisions for a commercial bank to offer loans and the decisions for a non-finance firm to raise debt and so on are all made without solid foundations.

Although millions of related decisions are made every day in the world, most of them have to be made intuitively rather than under the guidance of some reliable financial methods or models. The following chapters reveal that some of the prevailing financial methods or models have fundamental defects in logic. Financial studies after Gordon, Sharpe, Modigliani and Miller gradually turn to empirical researches, which focus on explanation of past sample data rather than finding solutions to important financial problems. Therefore, these fundamental problems remain unsolved for decades. Obviously, solving these fundamental problems is helpful for strengthen the mansion of financial theory and helpful for decision-making in practice. This is the intention of this book.

The rest of this book is arranged as following. Chapters 2 and 3 deal with the fundamental problem (1) and (2) listed in last section. Chapter 2 reveals that a prevailing way to consider expected returns is not correct; we do not even know the perpetual grow rate is positive or negative; hence a currently wide-spread application of DCF is just something for show. Chapter 3 builds a series of new valuation models based on a brand new criterion aimed at overcoming the defects of current DCF, and further derives a series of theoretical ratio models. Chapter 4 examines the prevailing methods to determine a discount rate, including the application of CAPM and the variants, and proves again that the current application of DCF is just something for show. Further, this chapter builds a series of new models and methods to consider properly risk in valuation, including models of certainty equivalent, total risk premium, etc. Chapter 5 examines prior theories and models concerning capital structure, and builds a series of new models to trade-off the cost and benefit of debt financing and finally solves the problem of optimal capital structure.

Chapter 2
Does a Positive Perpetual Growth Rate Exist?

As discussed in Chap. 1, asset future risk and returns determine its current value. The so called risk is the uncertainty of the future returns. Thus the asset return forecast is very important for asset valuation and financial decisions. It is too difficult or inefficient to forecast asset returns from year to year. A more reasonable way is to forecast an average growth rate, so that all future (annual) returns can be derived based on a current (annual) return and the average (annual) growth rate. This is the convention in finance so far.

2.1 Average Annual Growth Rate Revisit

Forecast is a tough task. Asset returns (earnings or cash flows) forecast is not an exception. Although forecast is not the theme or core function of finance, finance is responsible for the forecast feasibility of the variables incorporated in its theories and models. This should be the minimum requirement or standard for financial theories and models, because finance as an independent science is decision or application oriented.

It is not feasible to forecast asset future returns year by year. A wiser choice is to forecast an average annual growth rate extended into the future. Combining this forecasted average annual growth rate and a (normalized) current return, one can derive all future returns of the asset. This has become a convention since the early days of finance as an independent science. The average annual growth rate is often referred to as a constant growth rate.

When we use an average annual growth rate in a financial model, an inevitable question is: how long is the time horizon considered for averaging out the growth rate. This is actually determined by the valuation method chosen. Within the context of DCF method, an asset value is the sum of the present values of its all future cash flows. As lifespan varies across assets, the infallible choice of time horizon is the infinite future. Hence the constant growth rate is the average annual growth rate over an infinite time horizon, which is usually called a perpetual growth rate in current financial community.

For example, Gordon (1962) derives a stock valuation model[1] with such a perpetual growth rate as an independent variable. Gordon's model takes the form:

$$p = \frac{D_0(1+g)}{k-g} = \frac{D_1}{k-g} \qquad (2.1)$$

Where D_0 is the dividend paid per share in current year, $D_1 = D_0(1+g)$ is the estimated dividend per share in next year, k is the market (investors) required rate of return on this stock, and g is the estimated constant perpetual growth rate of dividend.

Equation 2.1 is referred to as Gordon growth model or constant growth model in finance community. This model is widely used for stock valuation as well as for other asset valuation because of its multiple advantages, which include at least:

(1) Simplicity

Simplicity is necessary for a model to be feasible in application. As an application-oriented science, finance should care about the simplicities of its theory and model. The Gordon growth model (referred to as Gordon model hereafter) is an ideal model in such a sense. The (independent) variables taken into account are not much. The form of the model is very simple. In addition, its logic or derivation process is very easy to understand.

Viewing dividends as the cash flows of stock, the dividend in year 1, year 2, ..., year t, ... is $D_1 = D_0(1+g)^1$, $D_2 = D_0(1+g)^2, \ldots, D_t = D_0(1+g)^t, \ldots$ respectively. Value a stock by add the present values of all its future dividends,

$$P = \frac{D_0(1+g)^1}{(1+k)^1} + \frac{D_0(1+g)^2}{(1+k)^2} + \cdots \frac{D_0(1+g)^t}{(1+k)^t} \cdots \qquad (2.2)$$

Thus,

$$p\frac{(1+g)}{(1+k)} = \frac{D_0(1+g)^2}{(1+k)^2} + \frac{D_0(1+g)^3}{(1+k)^3} + \cdots \frac{D_0(1+g)^t}{(1+k)^t} \cdots \qquad (2.3)$$

Equation 2.2 minus Eq. 2.3,

$$P\left[1 - \frac{(1+g)}{(1+k)}\right] = \frac{D_0(1+g)^1}{(1+k)^1} \qquad (2.4)$$

Then,

$$P = \frac{D_0(1+g)}{k-g} = \frac{D_1}{k-g}$$

---

[1] We will discuss it further in Chap. 3 [1].

2.1 Average Annual Growth Rate Revisit

(2) Soundness

Finance as a science or financial theory should be correct exactly in concept. The Gordon model and the variables incorporated are all correct exactly in concept. For instance, g in the model is a perpetual growth rate rather than an average annual growth rate over any finite time horizon, which is in line exactly with the concept of DCF method. In addition, the asset value increases as the future return (determined by the D and g) goes up and decreases as the future risk (incorporated in the k) goes up, which is in line with the axiom of asset value determination. As discussed in Chap. 1, this axiom should be the basic standard to build and to judge a financial or valuation model.

The perpetual growth rate of returns has been a necessary variable in financial analyses and asset valuations since the Gordon model which is widely used to value stock as well as other assets. Understandingly, the principle of value determination is the same for various assets, and the only different is the content of the cash flows or returns. For stock valuation, it is dividend or earnings; for firm valuation, it is operating cash flows or free cash flows.

2.2 Arithmetic or Geometric Average Growth Rate

Again, finance as a science or financial theory should be correct exactly in concept. There are two basic ways to obtain an average growth rate: arithmetic averaging and geometric averaging. We thus should make sure which is correct to choose.

Growth means the value change of a variable across times or periods. Let V_t and V_{t-1} to be the value of a variable in year t and year t-1 respectively, assuming they occur at the end of the year; define V_t/V_{t-1} as the growth factor of the variable in year t. Hence the growth rate in year t is "$V_t/V_{t-1}-1$". Use AAG and GAG to represent the arithmetic average growth rate and the geometric average growth rate respectively. Then,

$$\text{AAG} = \frac{V_1/V_0 + V_2/V_1 + V_3/V_2 + \cdots + V_n/V_{n-1}}{n} - 1 \qquad (2.5)$$

$$\text{GAG} = \left(\frac{V_1}{V_0} \times \frac{V_2}{V_1} \times \frac{V_3}{V_2} \times \cdots \times \frac{V_n}{V_{n-1}}\right)^{\left(\frac{1}{n}\right)} - 1 = \left(\frac{V_n}{V_0}\right)^{\left(\frac{1}{n}\right)} - 1 \qquad (2.6)$$

Consider an example. Investor W buys a stock today at a price of 100. The price goes up to 150 at the end of year 1 and goes down to 100 at the end of year 2. Then, what is the average annual growth rate of the stock price? Our intuition tells us that the average annual growth rate is 0 %. However, if we calculate it based on Eqs. 2.5 and 2.6, the average annual growth rate is 8.33 % and 0 % respectively.

This demonstrates that the GAG is correct, whereas the AAG is not. Please note that the annual growth rate under GAG is affected only by the beginning value and final value of the variable, and independent of all the intermediate ups and downs. Obviously, when the growth rate of every year is indeed constant, GAG is equal to AAG; otherwise, GAG is less than AAG. If the standard deviation of the yearly growth rates is SD, the relationship between AAG and GAG is:

$$(1 + AAG)^2 = (1 + GAG)^2 + SD^2 \tag{2.7}$$

Actually, the arithmetic averaging is more suitable for measuring the absolute growth, i.e., the annual growth in value; whereas the geometric averaging is more suitable for measuring the relative growth, i.e., the annual growth rate. In other words, using AAG' to represent the average annual absolute growth, Eq. 2.5 should be rewritten as:

$$AAG' = \frac{(V_1 - V_0) + (V_2 - V_1) + (V_3 - V_2) + \cdots + (V_n - V_{n-1})}{n} = \frac{V_n - V_0}{n} \tag{2.8}$$

Based on Eq. 2.8, the average annual absolute growth of the stock price is 0 dollars, which is in line with our intuition. Similarly, the annual absolute growth under Eq. 2.8 (AAG') is also affected only by the beginning value and final value of the variable, and independent of all the intermediate ups and downs. Therefore when we use average growth rate, keep it in mind that it should be a geometric average. This is also in line with the convention of compounding growth and compounding discounting in finance.

2.3 ZZ Growth Paradox

Mathematically, the Gordon model or Eq. 2.1 requires that $k > g$. This is often mentioned or stressed in finance textbooks. However, a neglected but very important question is: does a positive perpetual growth rate exist?

Surprisingly, the answer is "No". There is actually no positive perpetual growth rate for any firm. If we define it as a constant (average) growth rate extended into the infinite future, what we obtain can only be a negative growth rate.

The reasoning is very simple. No firm can live forever. Expected returns in any form (accounting earnings, operating or free cash flows, and dividends on stock, etc.) will be zero over a long enough time or infinite future, because a firm will surely go bankrupt or disappear given such a long enough time!

Bankruptcy or disappearance is the inevitable destination of every firm in reality. Even being absorbed into another firm via purchase and acquisition, a firm finally cannot escape from disappearance together with the buyers. How strong and brilliant are the corporate behemoths like Barings Bank (1762–1995), Lemon Brothers (1950–2008), Eastman Kodak (1880–2012), etc. used to be? But where are they today?

2.3 ZZ Growth Paradox

Most of firms in the world so far are less than 1000 years old. Unfortunately, the average lifespan of leading US companies listed in the S&P 500 index has decreased by more than 50 years in the last century, from 67 years in the 1920 s to just 15 years today, according to Professor Richard Foster from Yale University [2].

Obviously, it needs not an infinite time for a firm to devalue to zero. Based on Eq. 2.6, in a long enough but finite time horizon, i.e., before n → ∞, the value of returns will goes from a positive number (V_0) to a number close to zero (V_n → 0). This implies that (V_n/V_0) < 1, hence (V_n/V_0)$^{(1/n)}$ < 1. GAG or geometric average growth rate thus can only be negative.

The prevailing convention in finance (practical research and theoretical research), however, is to assume (or forecast or estimate) a positive perpetual growth rate when valuing an asset with the Gordon model. This implies probably that most (if not all) of the applications of Gordon model are just for show. Obviously, when one of the variables input of the model are wrong about positive or negative, it is enough to result to an intolerant mistake. We thus cannot expect a correct result based on such inputs.

An explanation for such a convention is that it is helpful for simplifying the calculation. The returns of a firm are likely to increase for a short or long time and decline thereafter. Within the context of DCF valuation, cash flows in far away are less important because of the discounting. Thus, making a mistake over the declining period (treating a negative growth as a positive growth) will not affect the valuation result too much. This explanation is obviously not convincing. Simplification is not a good excuse for changing the sign of growth rate from negative to positive. Put it another way, we can simplify the calculation while keeping the growth rate negative rather than changing it to a wrongly positive.

There is another convention in applying Gordon model, which is discounting the returns of an asset over years in near future and applying Gordon model for the returns thereafter with a constant positive growth rate. Although most financial researchers are used to such a way, it is real wrong to assume a constant positive growth rate in such circumstances, because the far future (after the near future years) is more likely to grow negatively.

Anyway, it is rather difficult for current finance community to accept the negative long term or perpetual growth rate. In addition, the valuation result with a negative growth rate will be unacceptable lower than that with a positive growth rate.

Consider an acceptable stock with a perpetual growth rate of dividend of 7 % and a discount rate of 10 %. If we suppose the current dividend (year 0) of this stock is 1 dollar, based on the Gordon model, value of a share will be:

$$p = \frac{D_0(1+g)}{k-g} = \frac{1 \times (1+7\%)}{10\% - 7\%} = 35$$

This is the prevailing valuation.

Now let us take the lifespan of the firm into account. Assume this is a typical firm listed in the S&P 500 index, and its life expectancy is 41 years (= 67 × 50 % + 15 × 50 %). Assuming the dividend at the end of year 41 is zero will result in a −100 % annual growth rate of dividend. To make our calculation more meaningful, let us assume a dividend at the end of year 41 is something close to zero, say, 1/1000000 dollars. Thus, the average annual growth rate is:

$$\text{GAG} = \left(\frac{1/1000000}{1}\right)^{\left(\frac{1}{41}\right)} - 1$$
$$= 0.7139 - 1 = -28.6\%$$

Take the -28.6% (an average annual growth rate over 41 years) approximately as the perpetual growth rate, based on the Gordon model, the share value,

$$p = \frac{D_0(1+g)}{k-g} = \frac{1 \times (1 - 28.6\%)}{10\% + 28.6\%} = 1.85$$

Obviously, the valuation difference between 35 and 1.85 is too large to be reconciled by prevailing financial wisdom. The most important and most urgent problem, however, is not to explain the difference, but to judge which one is correct, or which one is more correct.

Unfortunately, it is rather difficult to answer such a "simple" question. On one hand, the valuation result of "1.85", which is 95 % lower than the "normal valuation" result of 35, is too low for most people to accept. On the other hand, the valuation based on a positive perpetual growth rate seems specious, because no firms will grow positively forever; the average growth rate, based on correct concept and logic, can only be negative.

The plausible negative growth rate thus brings us a dilemma: we can hardly accept a negative perpetual growth rate; but the perpetual growth rate can only be negative in logic. As such a dilemma is hard to be explained or solved; we refer to it as the "ZZ growth paradox". It seems urgent, because the long-term or perpetual growth rate is an inevitable variable in many financial and valuation models. Challenging by the ZZ growth paradox, many prevailing financial models and analyses seem on the verge of collapse.

The challenge from the ZZ growth paradox, however, is not as terrible as it seems to be at the first sight. We will further our discussion to reveal the implications of the ZZ growth paradox to valuation and finance, rather than to persuade readers to accept the negative growth rate. The numerical examples in the following discussions should not be regarded as practical guidance, but just for stimulating fundamental rethinking, and hopefully such rethinking can lead to more insights beyond the existing financial theory.

2.4 Bankruptcy Probability and Firm Life

The ZZ growth paradox reminds us that when valuing an asset or just estimating the growth of the asset returns, asset life should be considered as an important factors. Assets or stocks have finite lifespan, because firms will go bankrupt for sure someday in the future. Let us explore the bankruptcy probability and the firm life determination in this section based on Moody's data of actual corporate accumulated default rates.

2.4 Bankruptcy Probability and Firm Life

Moody's often publishes actual accumulated default rates over one year to ten year's periods for various rated firms, as shown in Table 2.1.

Please note that Moody's "default" by definition is different from "bankruptcy". In academic concepts and common understanding, bankruptcy means the end of the firm life hence vanishing of the stock value. Moody's default includes the bankruptcy as well as some situations of financial distress. This implies that the actual cumulative bankruptcy probability is lower than the corresponding percentage in Table 2.1.

Let b represent the bankruptcy probability over one year, hence (1-b) is the survival probability over one year. Thus the probability that a firm will survive over

Table 2.1 Moody's historical average cumulative default rates: 1970-2006

years	1	2	3	4	5	6	7	8	9	10
Aaa (%)	0.000	0.000	0.000	0.026	0.099	0.172	0.250	0.334	0.424	0.520
Aa (%)	0.008	0.019	0.042	0.106	0.177	0.260	0.343	0.415	0.463	0.522
A (%)	0.021	0.095	0.220	0.344	0.472	0.614	0.759	0.925	1.105	1.286
Baa (%)	0.181	0.506	0.929	1.433	1.937	2.449	2.956	3.448	4.013	4.633
Ba (%)	1.203	3.222	5.568	7.953	10.207	12.226	13.992	15.690	17.371	19.095
B (%)	5.235	11.298	17.044	22.054	26.791	30.976	34.762	37.972	40.908	43.322
Caa-C (%)	19.466	30.509	39.731	46.935	52.659	56.841	59.965	63.289	66.359	69.251

Source Richard Cantor, David T. Hamilton, Jennifer Tennant [3]

Table 2.2 Expected firm life and cumulative bankruptcy probability

	Firm ratings						
	Aaa	Aa	A	Baa	Ba	B	Caa-C
5-year cumulative default rates (Moody's) (%)	0.099	0.177	0.472	1.937	10.207	26.791	52.659
5-year cumulative bankruptcy probability (%)	0.050	0.089	0.236	0.969	5.104	13.396	26.330
One-year bankruptcy probability (%)	0.010	0.018	0.047	0.194	1.042	2.835	5.928
Constant one-year bankruptcy probability (%)	0.510	0.515	0.534	0.630	1.181	2.347	4.357
Expected firm life[a] (years)	196.00	194.07	187.10	158.69	84.66	42.61	22.95
10-year CBP[b] (%)	4.986	5.035	5.218	6.126	11.203	21.138	35.949
20-year CBP (%)	9.724	9.816	10.164	11.876	21.152	37.808	58.975
50-year CBP (%)	22.567	22.764	23.506	27.100	44.795	69.498	89.220
100-year CBP (%)	40.041	40.346	41.486	46.855	69.524	90.696	98.838
200-year CBP (%)	64.049	64.414	65.761	71.756	90.712	99.134	99.986
500-year CBP (%)	92.250	92.445	93.140	95.761	99.737	99.999	100.00
1000-year CBP (%)	99.399	99.429	99.529	99.820	99.999	100.00	100.00

[a] According to Queuing Theory, The expected firm life is simply the reciprocal of the corresponding constant one-year bankruptcy probability
[b] CBP = cumulative bankruptcy probability

n consecutive years is $(1-b)^n$. So the cumulative bankruptcy probability B over n consecutive years is:

$$B = 1 - (1-b)^n \qquad (2.9)$$

Considering the difference between the bankruptcy and the default, take half of the default rates in Table 2.1 as the cumulative bankruptcy probabilities. To reduce the uncertainty of the actual bankruptcy probabilities in any one year, we can work out the average one-year bankruptcy probability based on the five-year cumulative bankruptcy probability (column 6 of Table 2.1)[2] by using Eq. 2.9 inversely, as shown in row 1–3 of Table 2.2.

To calculate the cumulative bankruptcy probabilities over various time horizons in the future, we need a constant one-year bankruptcy probability. The average one-year bankruptcy probability in row 3 of Table 2.2 cannot be used for such a purpose, because it is under the assumption that the firm keeps its original rating unchanged in the future. Therefore, this average one-year bankruptcy probability should be adjusted further according to the likelihood of rating shift[3] of the firm in the future, because the firm's rating shift will affect the one-year bankruptcy probability significantly.

To make things simple, assume any year in the future, a firm is 70 % likely to keep its rating in the previous year and 5 % likely to shift to every other rating.[4] Under such an assumption, the constant one-year bankruptcy probabilities of various rated firms can be worked out as shown in row 4 of Table 2.2. Based on such constant one-year bankruptcy probabilities, we further derive the life expectancies of various rated firms and cumulative bankruptcy probabilities over various time horizons, shown in row 5–12 of Table 2.2.

To be simple, refer to firms rated from Aaa to A as A firms, firms rated from Baa to B as B firms and firms rated from Caa to C as C firms. In Table 2.2, expected life of A firms is around 190 years; expected life of B firms is 50–150 years; expected life of C firms is under 30 years. Over 50 % of B and C firms cannot avoid bankruptcy in 100 years. Most (92–100 %) firms cannot avoid bankruptcy in 500 years. In a time horizon of 1000 years, the cumulative bankruptcy probability is over 99 % even for the Aaa firms. This reflects the reality to a large extent, since we rarely see a firm living over 1000 years.[5]

---

[2] Choice of other column will not change the results too much. Note that most of the standpoints here related to the negative growth rate are logically sound. The calculations are mainly for illustrative purposes, and some impreciseness in assumptions or data will not hurt the conclusions. Therefore, we prefer the simpler assumption or data processing for simplifying the illustrating as long as it is not far from reality.

[3] Although we need not to stress on the preciseness, we do consider the significant differences or changes in various concepts and calculations.

[4] Note that there are 7 ratings listed here, and 70 % × 1 + 5% × 6 = 100 %, and adjusting downward of the "70 %" and consequently adjusting upward of the "5 %" will increase the constant one year bankruptcy probabilities of A firms and decrease the constant one year bankruptcy probabilities of C firms.

[5] According to the survey of O'Hara (2002), only 3 companies have been living over 1000 years so far.

2.5 Is Bankruptcy Loss Incorporated into Discount Rate?

Since the negative growth rate is hard to be accepted, we try to seek some reasons for the positive growth rate in this section. First, is it possible that the bankruptcy risk is already incorporated into the discount rate k, so we do not need to take bankruptcy into account when we estimate the growth rate? If it is true, the positive perpetual growth rate is possible.

In finance, risk is uncertainty of future returns. The bankruptcy expectation actually has double effects. One is reducing the returns and the other is increasing the total risk. The former comprises expected losses resulting from suspension of operations due to bankruptcy, as represented by a certain negative growth rate. The later is the uncertainty of bankruptcy and can be represented by the increase of the discount rate k.

As discussed above, firms cannot escape from bankruptcy. When the bankruptcy occurs, a firm normally left nothing to its stock value. Therefore, viewing from the shareholders point at any time before the actual bankruptcy, the expected bankruptcy loss is simply the total value of the equity. Viewing from the whole firm point, the expected bankruptcy loss is even larger as it may also include the loss of the debt-holders. For the purpose of stock valuation, it is correct to define the (expected) bankruptcy loss as the current value of the stock or equity.

Theoretically, the uncertainty of bankruptcy should definitely be factored into the required or expected rate of return, k. In practice, however, the convention is to estimate k using the capital assets pricing model (CAPM) or some of its modifications, such as the Fama/French Three Factor Model[6] In determining the risk premium of a stock, CAPM and its modifications only account for systematic risk, as represented by the betas in the models, and assume non-systematic risks of all the individual stocks will offset each other in a rationally or perfectly diversified portfolio investment.

On the other hand, results of various researches[7] demonstrate that bankruptcy risk is not rewarded by higher returns and there are ongoing debates upon whether or not bankruptcy risk belongs to systematic risk. Therefore, the discount rate k derived from CAPM accounts at most for bankruptcy risk, but definitely does not account for expected bankruptcy loss. Risk is uncertainty. As bankruptcy will occur for sure over a long enough time horizon, the 100 % possible bankruptcy loss is virtually a negative return rather than a risk. Even if the bankruptcy risk is incorporated into the discount rate, the final expected loss still has to be incorporated into the growth rate. Hence a negative growth rate is unavoidable.

Nevertheless, it is interesting to calculate how much the conventional discount rate should be adjusted to account for all risks as well as the expected bankruptcy loss and thereby to justify a conventional positive perpetual growth rate. Let's just do that based on the example assumed in Sect. 2.3, in which the discount rate is 10 %, and current dividend is 1 dollar, with a positive perpetual growth rate of 7 %.

---

[6] See Fama Eugene F. and French Kenneth R. [4, 5].
[7] See among others, Dichev, Ilia D [6].

Firstly, we assume the bankruptcy loss is incorporated into the negative growth rate and all the risks, including bankruptcy risk, are included in the discount rate k. As shown in the Sect. 2.3, the valuation result is 1.85.

The Gordon model implies,

$$k = [D_0(1+g)]/p + g \tag{2.10}$$

Now, based on the share value of 1.85 dollars and using the "conventional perpetual growth rate" of 7 % instead of the negative growth rate of -28.6 %, we can find an implied k which accounts for not only the relevant risks but also the bankruptcy loss:

$$k = [D_0(1+g)]/p + g = 1(1+7\%)/1.85 + 7\% = 64.84\%$$

Thus, for a typical firm, if we incorporate the expected bankruptcy loss into the discount rate k, it should be as high as 64.84 %. This "surprising high discount rate" further confirms that conventional discount rates of around 10 % really have not accounted for bankruptcy loss. Hence the positive perpetual growth rate has no chance to be justified.

Viewing from a stand point, a firm has two kinds of risk: one is operating risk, shown as the fluctuations of earnings and value of the firm along with the change of the conditions within and outside the firm; another is bankruptcy risk, shown as the suspension of operation once the firm's value at the debt maturity falls below its debt book value. If a firm has no debt in its capital mix, it has only operating risk and has no bankruptcy risk.

Therefore, it is important to distinguish the bankruptcy cost and bankruptcy loss. The bankruptcy cost is corresponding to debt financing and bankruptcy risk. We will discuss it further in the fifth chapter for solving the problem of optimal capital structure. The bankruptcy loss is corresponding to the firm's total risk, including operating risk and bankruptcy risk. Obviously, for stock valuation, we should consider all risks rather than only bankruptcy risk, i.e. we should consider the bankruptcy loss rather than bankruptcy cost. If we forget the expected bankruptcy loss in valuing a stock, whether bankruptcy risk (bankruptcy cost) is incorporated into the discount rate is actually not so important, because the bankruptcy loss is much bigger in size than the bankruptcy cost.

2.6 The Implied Perpetual Growth Rate

A natural way to estimate a perpetual growth rate is using Gordon growth model inversely based on the price data of the relevant asset or its comparables.

$$g = \frac{Pk - D_0}{P + D_0} \tag{2.11}$$

The growth rate derived based on Eq. 2.11 is referred to as implied perpetual growth rate. For example, analysts often derive the perpetual growth rate of a

2.6 The Implied Perpetual Growth Rate

stock based on the implied growth rates of comparable stocks. This is virtually wrong because, it actually has a strict premise that the prices of the comparable stocks used as the estimation base must be correct, i.e. the comparable stocks must be fair-priced in the market.

Theoretically, we cannot judge a stock or an asset is fairly priced or not before we value it based on convincing method and model as well as reliable inputs. It is easy to work out an implied growth rate based on Eq. 2.11, but it is not easy to determine whether it is right, because it is not easy to make sure whether the comparable assets are fair-valued in the market. Since stocks are mispriced in the market more often than not, it is rather difficult to find a correct or reliable implied growth rate.

There is another common way to estimate the perpetual growth rate, which is based on a stock index. Based on Standard & Poors 500 over 1960–2007, for instance,[8] we may work out an average rate of return (viewed as discount rate) of 10 % or so and an average growth rate (viewed as perpetual growth rate) of 7 % or so. The discount rate of 10 % and growth rate of 7 % are so "typical" that they are often used in financial classes and textbooks to exemplify the DCF valuations and calculations.

This is virtually wrong at least in two aspects.

On one hand, every specific stock relies on the life of the relevant firm. The life of any firm is much different from that of any stock index. A stock index survives when failed firms replaced by new firms, whereas the stock of the failed firm and its related cash flows are worthless. The growth rate derived this way is just a growth rate of a stock index over a finite time horizon. The problem is: the growth rate of a stock index cannot represent that of a stock, because the life of a stock index is much different from that of a stock. Even the life of typical or average stock is much shorter than that of a stock index.

On the other hand, forgetting the difference between the life expectancy of a stock index and a specific stock, i.e., assuming both a stock and the index have infinite life and that the stock is a typical stock in the index, this is still not correct in most circumstances as a way to obtain a growth rate for a stock, because it requires the index data must be correct, which implied that all stocks in the index were always fairly priced in the market, or the stocks being over priced is always cancel out exactly by the stocks being under priced. This is not possible. Thus, the growth rate derived this way is hardly to be right.

---

[8] Based on the data of Aswath Damodaran (2008), yearly data of the S&P 500 from 1960 to 2007 (http://pages.stern.nyu.edu/~adamodar/New_Home_Page/datafile/spearn.htm), the author find that the compound annual growth rate (capital gain) of the S&P 500 was 7.12 %, the average annual dividend yield was 3.26 % and the average annual total return was 10.38 %.

2.7 The Stage of Finance as a Science

More and more financial papers and books argue that our financial theory is so advanced that no new discoveries can be found without interdisciplinary studies. An interesting question is: which stage is our financial theory in over its life cycle?

If a subject is characterized as most fundamental problems remain unsolved, it must be in its initial stage or start phase. Obviously, the most urgent task for a subject in initial stage is to solve the fundamental problems within the field rather than to search for outside cooperation or interdisciplinary studies.

We find in last chapter that most of the fundamental problems in finance remain unsolved. Now, we further find that we even cannot make sure whether the perpetual growth rate, a very basic input in finance, is positive or negative!

We may say that Astronomy as a science now is in its advanced stage; but we have to say that Astronomy was in its initial stage 500 years ago, because most fundamental problems remained unsolved at the time. For instance, mankind could not make sure whether earth goes around sun or sun goes around earth. Now, in finance, the perpetual growth rate is not sure to be positive or negative!

Therefore, finance as a science (not as a practice) now is similar to Astronomy 500 years ago. This is not blamable. Just think that 500 years ago, in the time of Nicolaus Copernicus (1473–1543), how many years had been spent on the research of Astronomy. Comparably, how many years have been spent on the research of finance until today!

Thus, finance as a science is just in its initial stage or start phase. Nevertheless, finance is a science and we should try our best to solve the problems (especially the fundamental problems) one by one. The most important thing is that we should put our efforts on the right direction and go along the right way, so that we can really find effective and efficient solutions with correct and simple methods. Whether our efforts are on the right direction and right way is determined by the essential features of finance as a science, i.e. an application—oriented decision science based on valuation, as revealed in last chapter.

After all, we fail to justify a positive perpetual or long term growth rate. Combining with the conclusion of last chapter, we further find that finance as a science is just in its initial stage. Again, we do not necessarily agree with the negative growth rate, so we prefer to call the logic puzzle as "ZZ growth paradox". This paradox, unfortunately, is unavoidable for thinking and solving the unsolved fundamental financial problems, because the growth rate actually determines the future returns of an asset, which further determine the value of the asset. So, it is time for us to rethink fundamentally about finance.

References

1. Gordon MJ (1962) The savings investment and valuation of a corporation. Rev Econ Stat 44(1):37–51
2. Cantor R, Hamilton DT, Tennant J (2007) Confidence intervals for corporate default rates. Special Comment of Moody's, April 2007

References

3. Fama EF, French KR (1993) Common risk factors in the returns on stocks and bonds. J Financ Econ 33:3–56
4. Fama EF, French KR (1996) Multifactor explanations of asset pricing anomalies. J Financ 51:55–84
5. Dichev ID (1998) Is the risk of bankruptcy a systematic risk? J Financ 53:1131–1147
6. Ibbotson RG, Chen P (2003) Long-run stock returns: participating in the real economy. Financ Anal J 59(1)

Chapter 3
Valuation Based on Required Payback Period

We have known that risk and return determine asset value and finance as a science has not incorporated the returns well in valuation, since it is too difficult to make sure whether the perpetual growth rate (of annual returns) is positive or negative.

This chapter focuses on the problem of incorporating return in valuation, whereas next chapter focuses on the problem of incorporating risk in valuation. A brand new absolute valuation method abreast to the prevailing DCF method is introduced in this chapter, which hopefully can help us to step out of the dilemma of the ZZ growth paradox.

Similar to the Gordon growth model, while most of the discussions in this chapter seem concentrated on stock valuation, the models and principles revealed can actually be applied to other asset valuation as well. In other word, the discussions and conclusions in this chapter are concerning general valuation, including absolute and relative valuation.

3.1 Absolute Valuation and Relative Valuation

Assets can be valued with two basic approaches: absolute valuation and relative valuation. In absolute valuation, we value an asset based on its fundamentals, i.e. the risk and return of the asset; in relative valuation, we value an asset based on one or more value ratios or multiples of other similar or comparable assets, such as the price-earnings ratios of the stocks in the same industry or same sectors for stock valuation.

3.1.1 Absolute Valuation

The absolute valuation approach is equivalent to discounted cash flow (DCF) method so far. According to DCF method, value of an asset is the sum of all present values of its (forecasted or expected) future cash flows. The future cash flows represent the returns of the asset and vary from asset to asset in forms: dividends for stocks, coupons and the face value for bonds, and after-tax cash flows for a real project.

In DCF method, value of an asset is determined by two factors: future cash flows on the asset and discount rate used to discount the cash flows. The future cash flows represent the consideration for the asset return; and the discount rates represent the consideration for the assets risk, with higher rates for riskier assets and lower rates for safer assets. Therefore, the DCF method tallies with the value determination principle.

The DCF method hence is theoretically sound and widely used in academic and practical research. Applying to stock valuation, to be simple and feasible, assume or forecast an average annual growth rate of the future dividends, the model can be simplified as Gordon growth model (Gordon [1] hereafter referred to as Gordon model),

$$P = \frac{D_0(1+g)}{k-g} = \frac{D_1}{k-g} \qquad (3.1)$$

where P is the value of the stock; D_0 is dividend per share in current year; D_1 is dividend per share in next year; k is constant (or average) discount rate, defined as the market (investors) annual required rate of return on this stock; g is the (average) perpetual annual growth rate of the dividend of this stock.

We have focused on the discussion of the perpetual growth rate g and know that there is a growth paradox (ZZ paradox) against the application of Gordon model: it seems very difficult to make sure whether the perpetual growth rate is positive or negative. This implies that the widely applications of Gordon model are just something for show.

There are some practical improvements in applying the Gordon model, i.e. the two-stage or three-stage or even more-stage growth model. These improvements, though racking our brains, are virtually nothing but postponement the application of the Gordon model. Despite how many stages the future is divided into, the Gordon model have to be applied for the last stage to derive a "terminal value". However, once the Gordon model is used for the last stage, the perpetual growth rate g as an input cannot be avoided. Again, the growth paradox comes up: is the perpetual growth rate positive or negative after all?

Even worse, the Gordon model (including the two-stage or three-stage or even more-stage growth model) is widely used not only for stock valuation, but also for various assets (such as firm) valuations, such as the two-stage or three-stage free cash flow (to equity or to firm) model; its basic form (P = D1/(k − g)) becomes a necessary part for most (if not all) absolute valuations or DCF applications. In other words, there are seldom cases of DCF applications without the Gordon model.

Seems no way out? Do not give up! This chapter will provide a solution.

3.1.2 Relative Evaluation

As mentioned above, relative valuation values an asset based on some ratios or multiples of other comparable assets. It is hence referred to as ratio method.

3.1 Absolute Valuation and Relative Valuation

The ratios used in valuation are usually the ratios of asset price to a common variable. The common variable is often an important value driver for the relevant asset. The most common ratios in stock valuation include price-earnings ratio, price-book value ratio and price-sales ratio, which are referred to as P/E ratio, P/B ratio and P/S ratio respectively.

$$P/E = \text{share price} / \text{earnings per share} \quad (3.2)$$

$$P/B = \text{share price} / \text{book value per share} \quad (3.3)$$

$$P/S = \text{share price} / \text{sales per share} \quad (3.4)$$

where, earnings and sales are the earnings and sales in last 12 months or 1 year ended today respectively;[1] book value is the book value of net asset (equity) today.

Understandingly, when earnings or book value or sales is the most important value driver, we can choose P/E ratio, P/B ratio or P/S ratio to value the stock. For instance, we may choose P/E ratio to value stocks in manufacturing sector, or choose P/B ratio to value stocks in real estate sector, or choose P/S ratio to value stocks in retail sector. For a dot.com company, the number of user clicks may represents its value potential, so we can choose price-click ratio to value the stock.

The common variable is chosen based on the its importance as a value driver and its measurability. Once the common variable is determined, the next step is to choose some similar assets as comparable assets and calculate the related ratios of these comparable assets based on their current or historical data about prices and the common variables. Once the ratios of comparable assets obtained, the value of the asset can be derived by using the common variable of the asset under consideration times the (average) ratios of comparable assets. This is the common process for performing the relative valuation.

According to the discussion in last chapter, the growth rate implied in stock price is not necessarily correct, because the stock is not necessarily fairly priced. With the similar reasoning, the asset value derived via relative valuation is not necessarily correct, because the comparable assets are not necessarily fairly priced in the market hence their ratios are likely erroneous. This is true for relative valuation. In other words, relative valuation assumes that the market, on average, prices the comparable assets correctly.

While relative valuation may be able to identify the assets being relatively (but not absolutely) undervalued or overvalued in the market, it cannot indicate whether the market as a whole is undervalued or overvalued. Relative valuation thus is not a theoretical sound method in valuation. It is easy to misuse and

---

[1] There are a number of variants on the basic P/E ratio based upon how the price and the earnings are defined. For example, apart from the basic P/E ratio, the Forward P/E is also prevailing in stock market, which is defined as the ratio of the current share price to forecasted earnings per share next year. To focus our main intention of searching for solutions to fundamental financial problems, most of the reasoning in this chapter will be based on the basic P/E ratio. Of course, the conclusions are valid too for other P/E variants. For detail, see Aswath Damodaran [2]

manipulate. An obvious fact is that, the ratio varies from asset to asset; so that the average ratio used in valuation depends on the comparable assets selected. Even for the same comparable asset, the ratio varies from time to time, because the asset price fluctuates endlessly.

The allure of relative valuation is that it is simple and easy to use. It thus becomes the widely used valuation method in practice, especially in circumstances where a large number of comparable assets are traded in the market, and the market on average, prices these assets more or less correctly. Anyway, asset value derived via relative valuation may not be as reliable as that derived via absolute valuation. Since what this book focuses on is theoretical solutions to fundamental financial problems, we will not put too much attention on relative valuation. Now, the following question may make sense: what is the quantitative relationship between the relative valuation and the absolute valuation?

3.1.3 Option Pricing Valuation

Option pricing valuation, or contingent claim method, uses option pricing models to value assets with option characteristics. Most prevailing textbooks introduce it as the third valuation approach abreast to the traditional absolute valuation and relative valuation. This is not true. Option pricing valuation is actually a kind of absolute valuation, because it derives asset value based on the risk and return of the asset (the option).

3.1.3.1 Types of Option

Call Options and Put Options

There are two basic options: call options and put options. A call option (put option) gives the holder the right, but not the obligation, to buy (sell) a specific amount of a given underlying asset at a specified price (the strike price) during a specified period. Option buyers or holders pay for the option and then have the long positions with pure right on the option. The counterparties in the market receive the proceeds and then have the short positions with pure obligation on the option. When the investors with long positions want to exercise the options, investors with short positions have obligation to fulfill the exercising transaction. Figure 3.1 illustrates the payoffs of the four option positions.

Formal Options and Real Options

There are (call and put) options on various kinds of underlying assets, such as stock, commodity, currency, index, debt or bond, often referred to as stock option, commodity option, currency option, index option, debt or bond option

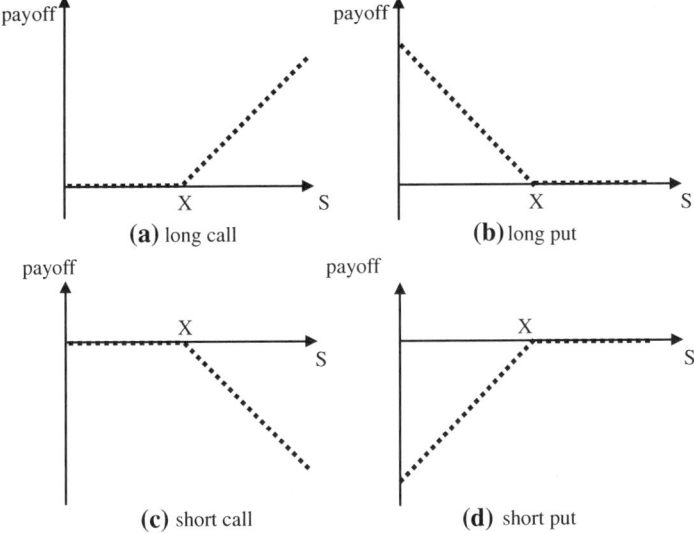

Fig. 3.1 The payoffs of the four option positions where, S = current price or value of the underlying asset. X = exercise price of the option. call = call option. put = put option

respectively. Apart from those formal options as derivatives in financial market, there are also some options related to some regular assets, such as a real project, a brand, a patent, etc. Such informal options are referred to as real options, since they are similar to the formal options for that they can also give the holders right but not the obligation to exercise the options in future. A lot of assets share option characteristics. Equity, for instance, can be viewed as a call option on the value of the underlying firm, with the strike price as the maturity value of the firm's debt and the maturity date as that of the firm's debt.

American Options and European Options

Options are different in terms of the exercise rule. Some options may only be exercised on expiration, known as European option; some options may be exercised on any trading day on or before expiration, known as American option; some options may be exercised only on specified dates on or before expiration, known as Bermudan option. "European", "American" and "Bermudan" here have no meaning of geographic area. Other things being equal, the value of an American option is likely larger than that of a Bermudan option, and the value of a Bermudan option is likely larger than that of a European option. However, the value differences among the three options are not so much as what they seem to be, since both American option and Bermudan option can be exercised only once. In many circumstances, the American option and Bermudan option are equal in value to the European option, because they may be not worth exercising before expiration.

In the Money and Out of the Money

As a contingent claim, at any given time before expiration, the payoff or intrinsic value of an option is either positive or zero. When the payoff or intrinsic value is positive, we say the option is in the money; when the payoff or intrinsic value is zero, we say the option is out of the money; as shown in Fig. 3.2. The point between "in the money" and "out of the money" is referred to as "at the money".

In Fig. 3.2, when $S = X$, an option is at the money, no matter it is call option or put option. When the market price of the underlying asset (S) is significantly (insignificantly) below the strike price (X), the call option is deep (slight) out of the money and the put option is deep (slight) in the money; When the market price of the underlying asset (S) is significantly (insignificantly) above the strike price (X), the call option is deep (slight) in the money and the put option is deep (slight) out of the money.

3.1.3.2 Option Pricing Model

Intrinsic Value and Time Value

The payoff is also referred to as intrinsic value of the option. The intrinsic value is the main part of the option value, but not the whole. Before expiration, there is another part of the option value, namely time value of option. Please note that the time value of option is totally different from the time value of money. The time value of option decrease as the option goes towards its maturity. The sum of the intrinsic value and time value is the option value, which is the benchmark for options to be fairly priced in market, as shown in Fig. 3.3.

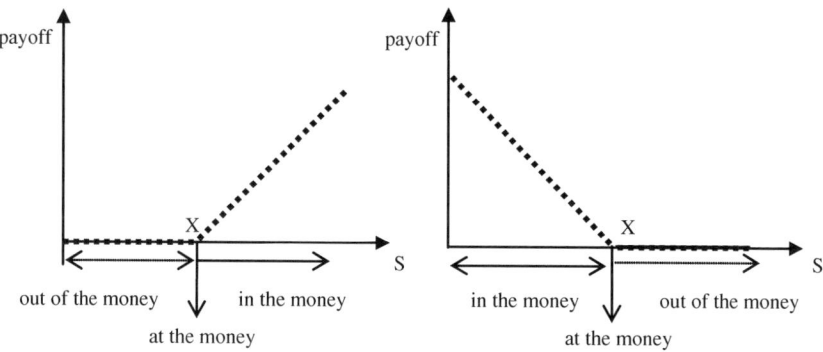

Fig. 3.2 In the money and out of the money options

3.1 Absolute Valuation and Relative Valuation

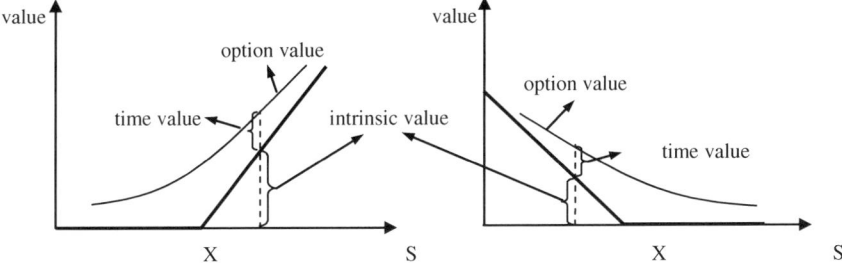

Fig. 3.3 Option value = intrinsic value + time value

Black–Scholes Model

Obviously, other things being equal, the deeper an option is in the money, the larger its value is. Out of the money options have only (positive) time value. While it is easy to calculate the intrinsic value or payoffs of an option, it is rather difficult to calculate the time value of an option. The exploration of option valuation had been lasted at least for 70 years until a reliable option pricing model published in 1973. The model is referred to as Black–Scholes model or Black–Scholes-Merton model:

$$c = SN(d1) - Xe^{-rT}N(d2) \tag{3.5}$$

$$p = Xe^{-rT}N(-d2) - SN(-d1) \tag{3.6}$$

Where, S is current price or value of the underlying asset; X is exercise price of the option; T is the maturity time (year) of the option; e^{-rT} is the present value coefficient under continuously compounding, i.e. the present value of 1 dollar received at the end of T year(s); N(d1) and N(d2) are the cumulative probability of a standard normal distribution with a z-score being d1 and d2 respectively; d1 and d2 can be derived with the following equations:

$$d1 = \frac{\ln(S/X) + (r + \sigma^2/2)T}{\sigma\sqrt{T}} \tag{3.7}$$

$$d2 = \frac{\ln(S/X) + (r - \sigma^2/2)T}{\sigma\sqrt{T}} = d1 - \sigma\sqrt{T} \tag{3.8}$$

where, σ is the volatility of the underlying asset, defined as the standard deviation (hence σ^2 is the variance) of annual returns on the underlying asset; ln (S/X) is the natural logarithm of (S/X), or the power to which e ($\approx$2.718281828…) would be raised to (S/X).

The Black–Scholes model is a ground-breaking innovation in finance. In 1997, Scholes and Merton were awarded the Nobel Prize in Economic Sciences for their work on option pricing.[2] Black–Scholes model solves the problem of option valuation to a large extent, although it is special for European options. Since value of American option is not much different from its European counterparty, the Black–Scholes model can be used to value most of the options including American and Bermudan options. While most real options are not strict European options, the valuation of these real options are usually not required to be precise. The Black–Scholes model thus can be used directly to value most real options.

In addition to the Black–Scholes model, the Cox, Ross and Rubinstein's binomial model (1979) and Monte Carlo simulation are also widely used as primary option pricing methods. As this book focuses on the solutions of unsolved fundamental financial problems, we will not further introduce these methods in detail. For more detail of option pricing model, see Black and Scholes [3], Merton [4], Cox, Ross and Rubinstein [5], and Hull [6].

3.1.3.3 Option Pricing in Valuation Spectrum

We know that value is the core of finance and that risk and return determine asset value. Further, cash flows (and earnings, etc.) are the specific form of return. The so-called risk is just the uncertainty of future cash flows. So we can say that an asset value comes from its future cash flows. There are two kinds of future cash flows in terms of the uncertainties. One is the future cash flow with uncertainty in size; the other is the future cash flow with uncertainty in emergence or existence. We refer to the former as volatile cash flows and the later as contingent cash flows. Therefore, value of an asset, such as a firm, comes from all its future cash flows, including volatile cash flows and contingent cash flows.

Obviously, the contingent cash flows like cash flows of options (exist when options are in the money; disappear when options are out of the money), no matter they are formal options or real options. Conventional valuation method or discounted cash flow approach is only correct for valuing volatile cash flows. For contingent cash flows from option-like assets, we cannot arbitrarily assume the cash flows will surely emerge or exist and discount them as what we do in valuing volatile cash flows. Therefore, to value option-like assets, we have to resort to option pricing model. Option-like assets can be found almost everywhere, since the basic option characteristics "with the right but not the obligation" simply means a kind of flexibility, which widely implied in most (if not all) assets.

The DCF method is somehow suitable to deal with the stable or volatile cash flows; whereas the option pricing model is somehow suitable to deal with the contingent cash flows. Therefore, the DCF method and option pricing method are complementary rather than competing approaches in absolute valuation. We may

---

[2] A Nobel Prize is not awarded posthumously but Fischer Black would undoubtedly have been a joint winner of the 1997 Nobel Prize for Economics had he lived. Black was unfortunately diagnosed with throat cancer in 1994 and died on 30 August 1995.

3.1 Absolute Valuation and Relative Valuation

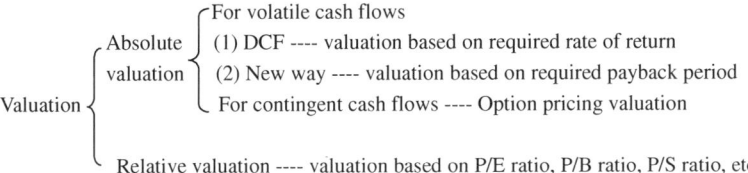

Fig. 3.4 The valuation approaches

have to resort both DCF method and option pricing method to complete the valuation of an asset when it has option characteristics. This implies that we can hardly value asset correctly without option pricing method. However, option pricing method is not as widely used as that of the DCF method. This may be an important reason that most of the fundamental financial problems remain unsolved. Figure 3.4 illustrates the valuation approaches and their relationships.

In Fig. 3.4, the second absolute valuation method for valuing volatile cash flows, i.e. valuation based on required payback period, is a brand new valuation method abreast to the DCF method. The rest part of this chapter will go into its details.

3.2 Cases When Current Absolute and Relative Valuation Invalid

The absolute valuation is currently equivalent to DCF method. As a matter of fact, this is a wide-spread misunderstanding. As indicated in last section, absolute valuation values an asset based on its risk and return. There may be one or more other alternatives to consider risk and return of an asset. While DCF method considers both risk and return of an asset, it is only one alternative as the absolute valuation.

Figure 3.4 indicates that, for valuing assets with volatile cash flows, there are at least two ways to consider the relevant risk and return. One is the valuation with the criterion of required rate of return (discount rate), which is the prevailing DCF method; the other is valuation with the criterion of required payback period, which is a brand new way in absolute valuation—again, it values asset based on its risk and return.

The original discovery on new method represents significant progress of a subject. As for today's finance, seeking for new absolute valuation method is not only necessary, but also very urgent, because the DCF method encounters serious crises. The current application of DCF method needs the aid of the Gordon model; but as revealed in last chapter, the Gordon model cannot get rid of the dilemma from the ZZ paradox. As a matter of fact, the crises are not limited to this. In addition to the inevitable paradox trouble, the result based on the Gordon model is too sensitive to some input values.

Consider the following two valuation examples.

Example (1): Given stock A, B and C, the perpetual growth rates of their dividends are 9 %, 9.9 % and 9.99 % respectively; their dividends per share next year are all 1 dollar; the market or investors required rate of return are all 10 %. How much are they in value today?

Example (2): Given tock D, E and F, the growth rate of their earnings per share over a foreseeable future period (about 15 years or so) are 10 %, 20 % and 30 % respectively; their current earnings per share are all 1 dollar; the market or investors required rate of return are all 10 %. How much are they in value today?

Both example (1) and (2) provide the data of risk and return. Now let us try to value the relevant stocks with some valuation method.

The data available of stock A, B and C are suitable to apply Gordon model, then:

$$P_A = \frac{1}{10\% - 9\%} = 100 \text{ (dollars)}$$

$$P_B = \frac{1}{10\% - 9.9\%} = 1000 \text{ (dollars)}$$

$$P_C = \frac{1}{10\% - 9.99\%} = 10000 \text{ (dollars)}$$

Value of B is 10 times of A, and value of C is 100 times of A, just because of the less than 1 % difference on their growth rates. We can regard A, B and C as actually just one stock, only that we "forecast" the growth rate as 9 % with an error of 0.9 % or 0.99 %. Since the g in Gordon model is the perpetual growth rate of dividends, i.e. the average annual growth rate over infinite time period, a forecasting error of 0.99 % is obviously inevitable. However, this inevitable and trivial error leads to a valuation bias of 10 times or even 100 times! This is obviously incredible and unacceptable.

Believe it or not, it is beyond the ability of human intelligence to forecast the average growth rate extended into infinite future, needless to say forecasting it with high precision or accuracy. Last chapter reveals that the perpetual growth rate is actually not sure to be positive or negative. Now, forgetting such a paradox trouble and assuming arbitrarily the perpetual growth rate can be positive, we still cannot save the Gordon model from palsy. After all, we find it is too difficult to work out a reasonable valuation result based on the Gordon model, because it requires a too precise perpetual growth rate.

Let's try further the example (2). Example (2) also provides the information of risk and return about stock D, E and F. The information of earnings instead of dividends is clearly more in line with practical investors' interests, because the earnings per share in any given year represent the total return on a share of stock in that year. Unfortunately, things now become even worse, since the Gordon model can do nothing about it.[3]

---

[3] Please note that "their earnings per share over foreseeable future period (such as about 15 years) are 10 %, 20 % and 30 % respectively" is a very realistic situation. For the DCF method, an asset value is the total present value of their future cash flows, including the cash flows over the foreseeable periods and those over the unforeseeable periods. But any assumption beyond the foreseeable period, such as cash flows are nothing or grow at a constant rate, etc. is conceptually unreliable and too arbitrary for valuation hence may result to a too big bias.

Among the prevailing financial tools, as the DCF method or Gordon model does not work, we have to resort to relative valuation or ratio method to solve the example (2). First of all, to apply the ratio method, such as the P/E ratio or P/B ratio or P/S ratio, we have to decide on which stocks are the comparables of stock D, E and F. Suppose it is easy to choose the right ratio and the right comparable stocks, there is still one tough question: ratios of the comparables at which dates can be the benchmark or valuation base?

This involves the fatal defect of ratio method or relative valuation. It is revealed in last section that relative valuation assumes all assets on average are fairly priced. However, that all assets on average are fairly priced can only be true for some time, because the prices of all assets and their average are all fluctuating over time. Therefore, if we believe that all assets on average are fairly priced at some times; we have to confess that all assets on average are not fairly priced at most (other) times.

After all, it cannot be clear that whether all assets on average are fairly priced. In other words, relative valuation or ratio method itself cannot prove that on which day or during which period, short or long, the comparable assets are fairly priced. While the risk and return of the comparable firms may be stable during a period, the prices of their stocks fluctuate every day and even every minute; the ratios thus vary across days or periods. Then, ratio over which period is right for valuing stock D, E and F?

Using average ratio over a short or long period instead of ratio on a single day cannot change the situation. The average ratio of one period is almost necessarily different from that of another period, and the differences are often not closely related with the changes of the risk and return of the firm. There may be a fair P/E or P/B or P/S ratio in a special past single minute or day, but the relative valuation approach itself cannot tell.

As such, it is not easy to obtain a convincing or reliable valuation result about stock D, E and F by using the relative valuation. The ratio method is most widely used in practice especially in valuation and investment, just because of its simplicity. However, if there is no effective way to determine a reliable or fair P/E, P/B or P/S ratio, its application, like that of the Gordon model, is inevitable to be something for show.

In sum, it seems to be the common or typical case when neither the DCF method nor the ratio method really works. This is really serious and urgent for our finance!

3.3 A New Absolute Valuation Method Based on Required Payback Period

Finance as a science is responsible to provide proper valuation methods and convincing valuation results, especially when the information about risk and return of an asset is given. The problems like the example (1) and (2) are so common, so typical and so simple in stock market as well as in financial market; financial theory is unshakably responsible to provide efficient model(s) to solve such kind of problems.

3.3.1 ZZ Growth Model

It seems impossible for the relative valuation to provide a theoretically sound model, since it does not consider synthetically the risk and return of an asset. So we should seek the way out via absolute valuation. As the only method so far in absolute valuation, discounted cash flow method is actually based on an investment criterion of required rate of return. There is another investment criterion, i.e. required payback period. A creative idea is that it may be possible to find a new valuation method based on such an investment criterion.

Suppose the current year's earnings per share is E, the average annual growth rate of the earnings in foreseeable future is g, then the annual earnings in the consecutive n years will be $E(1+g)^1$, $E(1+g)^2$, $E(1+g)^3$, ..., $E(1+g)^n$ respectively. Note that the earnings per share in any given year represent the total return on the stock in that year, and the value or price of the stock represents the initial investment. If the required payback period is n, then[4]:

$$P = E(1+g)^1 + E(1+g)^2 + E(1+g)^3 + \ldots\ldots + E(1+g)^n \quad (3.9)$$

Hence,

$$P(1+g) = E(1+g)^2 + E(1+g)^3 + \ldots\ldots + E(1+g)^{n+1} \quad (3.10)$$

3.10 minus 3.9,

$$gP = \left[(1+g)^n - 1\right](1+g)E \quad (3.11)$$

Hence,

$$P = \left[(1+g)^n - 1\right](1+g)E/g \quad (3.12)$$

Obviously, Eq. 3.12 is another absolute valuation model. Similar to Gordon model, Eq. 3.12 contains also a variable of growth rate g; I thus name Eq. 3.12 as ZZ growth model.[5] Please note that the g in the ZZ growth model is an average growth rate over a finite time horizon, which is different from that in the Gordon model. The ZZ growth model thus breaks away easily from the growth paradox trouble, because the average growth rate can certainly be positive in any foreseeable and finite period.

---

[4] Here we use the original concept of the payback period rather than the discounted payback period in many financial books and literature. The discounted payback period is a misleading concept because it incorporates two competing criteria: the required rate of return and the required payback period. In fact, the required payback period = 1/the required rate of return. Thus the application of the discounted payback period implies that the return requirement is satisfied twice in valuation or decision making. This makes no sense and is definitely wrong.

[5] The ZZ growth model cannot be abbreviated to "ZZ model", because there are other models invented by the author in the rest parts of this chapter and the following chapters.

3.3 A New Absolute Valuation Method Based on Required Payback Period

Understandingly, in the ZZ growth model, the foreseeable future, though no certainty requirement for its length, is supposed to be longer than the required payback period, so that the average annual growth rate of earnings g can extend beyond the required payback period n and the investor can get all his or her money back within the period of n years.

3.3.2 Solutions Based on ZZ Growth Model

Since the ZZ growth model is a fundamental innovation in finance and valuation, let us now test its power in solving practical problems like example (1) and (2). Note that in example (2), the required rate of return on D, E and F are all 10 % implies the required payback period are all 1/10 % = 10 years. The foreseeable period (about 15 years) is longer than the required payback period 10. Based on the ZZ growth model,

$$P_D = \left[(1 + 10\%)^{10} - 1\right](1 + 10\%)/10\% = 17.53 \text{ (dollars)}$$

$$P_E = \left[(1 + 20\%)^{10} - 1\right](1 + 20\%)/20\% = 31.15 \text{ (dollars)}$$

$$P_F = \left[(1 + 30\%)^{10} - 1\right](1 + 30\%)/30\% = 55.41 \text{ (dollars)}$$

Is the above valuation results yielded by the ZZ growth model reasonable or convinced? You can judge it based on your intuition or experience.

Let us further try the example (1).

The example (1) is designed for applying the Gordon model; we have to convert the data to fit the application of the ZZ growth model. As revealed in first section of this chapter, it is beyond human intelligence to forecast a perpetual growth rate. A reasonable inference is that the growth rates of 9 %, 9.9 % and 9.99 % are actually the growth rate over a foreseeable period. Since the growth rates are average growth rates over a finite time horizon, they can be positive; there is no paradox trouble now.

When a firm maintains its retention ratio,[6] the growth rate of earnings will be equal to that of the dividends. Although the growth rate of earnings may be higher or lower than the growth rate of dividends in any given year, the average growth rate of earnings over a very long period should be close or equal to the average growth rate of dividends. The growth rates of 9 %, 9.9 % and 9.99 % in example (1) thus can be viewed as the average growth rates of earnings of stock A, B and C over the foreseeable period (15 years or longer).

---

[6] Retention ratio indicates the percentage of a company's earnings that are not paid out in dividends but credited to retained earnings. The payout ratio is the amount of dividends the company pays out divided by the net income.
Retention Ratio = Retained Earnings/Net Income = 1 − Dividend Payout Ratio
Payout Ratio = Dividends Payout/Net Income = 1 − Retention Ratio.

To derive the data of initial earnings per share, we need further the retention ratios of the three firms. For the convenience of demonstration, assume they maintain the same retention ratio of 50 % over that foreseeable period. As their dividends in next year are all 1 dollar, their earnings per share in current year are:

$$E_A = 1/(1+9\%)/50\% = 1.8349 \text{ (dollars)}$$
$$E_B = 1/(1+9.9\%)/50\% = 1.8198 \text{ (dollars)}$$
$$E_C = 1/(1+9.99\%)/50\% = 1.8183 \text{ (dollars)}$$

Again, required rate of return 10 % implies that the required payback period is 10 years. Based on the ZZ growth model, the values of A, B and C are:

$$P_A = \left[(1+9\%)^{10} - 1\right](1+9\%) \times 1.8349/9\% = 30.39 \text{ (dollars)}$$
$$P_B = \left[(1+9.9\%)^{10} - 1\right](1+9.9\%) \times 1.8198/9.9\% = 31.72 \text{ (dollars)}$$
$$P_C = \left[(1+9.99\%)^{10} - 1\right](1+9.99\%) \times 1.8183/9.99\% = 31.86 \text{ (dollars)}$$

Comparing with the valuation results yielded by the Gordon model, that A, B and C are valued as 100 dollars, 1000 dollars and 10000 dollars respectively, the results above yielded by the ZZ growth model obviously make sense.

3.3.3 Comparison of Gordon Model and ZZ Growth Model

It seems easy for the ZZ growth model to solve the common and typical valuation problems that the Gordon model or DCF method and the ratio approach cannot. Since the Gordon model (including the two-stage and three-stage models) is used so widely, let us make a more detailed comparison of these two absolute valuation methods now.

We have discussed in last chapter that Gordon model has two advantages: theoretical soundness and simplicity. The ZZ growth model possesses both of them.

It is obvious that the ZZ growth model is simple in equation form and derivation process. The model takes only three key variables into account. Where, the E and g combine together as the consideration for the return of the asset; the n accounts for the risk of the relevant asset and n decreases as the risk increase. It even needs not discounting (see footnote 4 of this chapter), which is necessary for most (if not all) financial models.

As a fundamental axiom in finance, value (of an asset) increases with the increasing of the (expected) return and decreases with the increasing of the (expected) risk. Obviously, the ZZ growth model will result in a high value when the E and g are bigger (high return), and a low value when the n is smaller (high risk). Therefore, the ZZ growth model is completely in line with the fundamental financial axiom, i.e. it is theoretically sound.

3.3 A New Absolute Valuation Method Based on Required Payback Period

While the ZZ growth model possesses the same advantages as the Gordon model, it overcomes most of the shortcomings of the Gordon model.

Firstly, the application of both models needs its own condition. The Gordon model requires that the growth rate must be smaller than the discount rate, i.e. g < k. The condition of "g < k" restricts the application of the Gordon model seriously. For instance, it is hardly used to value high growth stocks. For the same reason, the valuation result is too sensitive to the growth rate. These restrictions deprive the basic feasibility of the model.

The ZZ growth model requires that the forecasting period should extend beyond the required payback period. This is just a reasonable requirement — analysts should do their best to forecasting into the far future, and poses no serious restriction for the application. As for the variable of growth rate, there is almost no restriction[7]; it can be any number greater than −100 %. The model thus can be used conveniently to value stocks in any sectors, including traditional sectors and high growth sectors.

Secondly, both models take three variables into account. According to the Gordon model, stock value is determined by dividends in current year D_0, the perpetual growth rate of the dividends g, and the investors' required rate of return (risk-adjusted discount rate) k. In theory, the estimations of the three variables should be correct over an infinite time horizon. Believe it or not, such requirements are actually beyond human intelligence.

According to the ZZ growth model, stock value is determined by earnings in current year E, the average growth rate of the earnings g, and the investors' required payback period (years) n. In theory, the estimations of the three variables should be correct over a finite time horizon. Such requirements are obviously more reasonable and feasible.

Earnings as a variable to represent return are more reliable and feasible to forecast than dividends. Even for the same finite time horizon, forecasting dividends and its growth is much more difficult than forecasting earnings and its growth, because the numbers of influential factors on dividends are at least one more — dividend policy.

A lot of firms employ residual dividend policy, under which they decide whether and how much to pay dividends in any year based on the earnings left after their investment demand got satisfied. As such, even the internal managers have no idea about the future dividends, needless to say the outsider analysts or investors.

In addition, the ZZ growth model is more realistic and practical because of the following facts: (1) Firms in reality all have limited life expectancies, rather than grow or live "forever". (2) Investors in reality have limited forecasting capability, and are not willing to base their valuations or decisions on the returns over an infinite period. (3) Comparing with the required rate of return, the required payback period is somehow more certain in intuition as a criterion for investment or decision, especially for immature investors.

---

[7] When g = 0, the ZZ growth model is: P = nE. .

After all, comparing with the Gordon model, the ZZ growth model has at least the following important advantages:

Firstly, the ZZ growth model avoids the paradox trouble and gains feasibility by adopting the new criterion of required payback period.

Secondly, the ZZ growth model gets rid off the unreasonable restrictions on the variable of growth rate and is flexible enough to value stocks in various sectors.

Thirdly, the result yielded by the ZZ growth model is properly sensitive rather than over sensitive to the growth rate and other variables incorporated, hence is reliable.

Before the ZZ growth model, there is never a valuation or pricing model based on the criterion of "required payback period". The absolute valuation models so far, traditional or modern, simple or sophistic, are all based on the criterion of "required rate of return" unexceptionally. In such a sense, the ZZ growth model is not only a brand new model, but also a brand new way abreast to the discounted cash flow approach. We will see further the problem-solving power of the ZZ growth model in the rest parts of this chapter.

Of course, there is no "perfect model" in this world. The ZZ growth model has its own drawback. It is well known that payback period as an decision criterion cannot account for the cash flows or returns beyond the payback period. So does the ZZ growth model. Because of this, the model is more suitable for the valuation of assets with future cash flows relatively well-distributed over years. For instance, it is more suitable for valuing assets like stocks, rather than bonds, etc., because the cash flows of bonds (including a big principal repayment) are usually not evenly distributed.

3.4 The Theoretical Ratio Models

We have seen the fatal defect of ratio method or relative valuation: it derives an asset value just based on the multiples of its comparable assets without a convincing judgment whether the comparables are fairly priced. Obviously, the effective remedy of such a defect depends on a theoretical ratio model. Let us try to find a way to build such model(s) now.

3.4.1 ZZ P/E Model

While P/E ratio is usually the ordinary P/E ratio defined as the current share price divided by earnings per share in most recent financial year, there are a number of variants on the basic P/E ratio in use, based upon how the price and the earnings are defined. One important variant is the forward P/E ratio, defined as the current share price divided by forecasted earnings per share next year. The P/E ratio in this chapter is referred to the ordinary P/E ratio unless indicated intentionally.

3.4 The Theoretical Ratio Models

A P/E model can be derived out based on the Gordon model via dividing the two sides of Eq. 3.1 by E:

$$P/E = \frac{D_0(1+g)/E}{k-g} = \frac{dr(1+g)}{k-g} \quad (3.13)$$

We refer to Eq. 3.13 as Gordon P/E model, where dr represents the average dividend payout ratio, which is equal to 1 minus the retention ratio.

Obviously, the Gordon P/E model is similar in form to the original Gordon model, hence carries on all the defects of the original Gordon model. As the most serious defect of the Gordon model, while the result of the Gordon P/E model is also too sensitive to the perpetual growth rate g, it is not sure whether the growth rate is positive or negative. Thus, this theoretical P/E model is not feasible.

Similarly, we can derive a theoretical P/E model based on the ZZ growth model via dividing the two sides of Eq. 3.12 by E:

$$P/E = \left[(1+g)^n - 1\right](1+g)/g \quad (3.14)$$

We refer to Eq. 3.14 as ZZ P/E model.[8] Needless to say, the ZZ P/E model possesses all the advantages of the ZZ growth model.

The ZZ P/E model has also another obviously advantage: it has only two variables—one less than that of the Gordon P/E model. According to the ZZ P/E model, a fair or theoretical P/E is determined by the growth potential (g) and risk (n) of the asset. The fair P/E increases as the growth potential increases and decreases as the risk increases because the n becomes smaller. These relationships definitely make sense.

Traditionally, investors and analysts believe that the appropriate P/E for most stock range around 10–30. While this may make some sense, may also confuses the investors and analysts when they confront nowadays' high tech or dot.com stocks. When you see in the market that "Google" is trading at a P/E around 500, how do you judge the price? Are you sure it is over-valued or under-valued? How can you work out (rather than guess carelessly) a relatively certain answer about such kind of questions?

There are rare effective tools suitable for solving these questions in current financial theory, although these questions are so common, so typical and so important for finance. That is one of the reasons why the related questions remain on-going debates. Applying the ZZ P/E model, however, it is easy to work out some reliable answers to the relevant questions based on responsible estimation on the earnings growth and the relevant risk of the stock.

For instance, if we believe that the average earnings growth rate of "Google" is around 100 % over a foreseeable period about 10–15 years, the investors' required payback period is 8 years based on its risk, its theoretical or fair P/E then is:

$$P/E = \left[(1+100\%)^8 - 1\right](1+100\%)/100\% = 510.00$$

---

[8] Note that when $g = 0$, the theoretical P/E model becomes: $P/E = n$.

The ZZ P/E model tells us that "Google" is not over-valued when its actual P/E is around 500 in the market so long as the inputs about the growth rate and required payback period are reliable. To get more intuition, Table 3.1 illustrates the theoretical or reasonable or fair P/Es based on the ZZ P/E model when the growth rate varies from −50 % to 100 % and required payback period varies from 5 to 10 years.

According to Table 3.1, if the earnings of a stock are expected to grow annually up to 10 % over more than 5–10 years, the theoretical P/E is less than 18. If the earnings are expected to grow at 20 % over more than 5–10 years, the theoretical P/E ranges between 9 and 30. If the earnings are expected to grow at 100 % over more than 5–10 years, the theoretical P/E is likely larger than 100, even larger than 1000 when the firm's businesses is really safe. If the earnings are expected to grow at −50 % over more than 5–10 years, the theoretical P/E is smaller than 1. These findings obviously make sense.

On the other hand, the traditional standard of 10–30 makes no sense, especially for those high growth stocks. As indicated by the ZZ P/E model, the fair P/E depends on the expected growth and required payback period. For a stock with high growth potential and low risk, a P/E of 1000 may not mean overvalued; however, if a stock has gloomy or dangerous future, a P/E of 5 may represent overvalued. It is clearly convenient to consider synthetically both the growth potential and risk in judging the fairness of a stock pricing with the ZZ P/E model.

Figure 3.5 shows the fair or theoretical P/E curves (FPC) based on the ZZ P/E model. X axis represents the expected growth rate and Y axis represents the fair P/E ratio. The 6 FPCs in Fig. 3.5 represent the required payback period of 5, 6, 7, 8, 9 and 10 years respectively. Every FPC goes up with the increasing of g, and

Table 3.1 The theoretical P/Es

n	g (%)							
	−50	−40	−30	−20	−10	0	10	20
5	0.97	1.38	1.94	2.69	3.69	5.00	6.72	8.93
6	0.98	1.43	2.06	2.95	4.22	6.00	8.49	11.92
7	0.99	1.46	2.14	3.16	4.70	7.00	10.44	15.50
8	1.00	1.47	2.20	3.33	5.13	8.00	12.58	19.80
9	1.00	1.48	2.24	3.46	5.51	9.00	14.94	24.96
10	1.00	1.49	2.27	3.57	5.86	10.00	17.53	31.15

n	g (%)							
	30	40	50	60	70	80	90	100
5	11.76	15.32	19.78	25.30	32.05	40.27	50.16	62.00
6	16.58	22.85	31.17	42.07	56.19	74.28	97.21	126.00
7	22.86	33.39	48.26	68.92	97.23	135.50	186.60	254.00
8	31.01	48.15	73.89	111.87	166.98	245.70	356.43	510.00
9	41.62	68.81	112.33	180.59	285.57	444.06	679.12	1022.00
10	55.41	97.74	170.00	290.54	487.17	801.11	1292.23	2046.00

3.4 The Theoretical Ratio Models

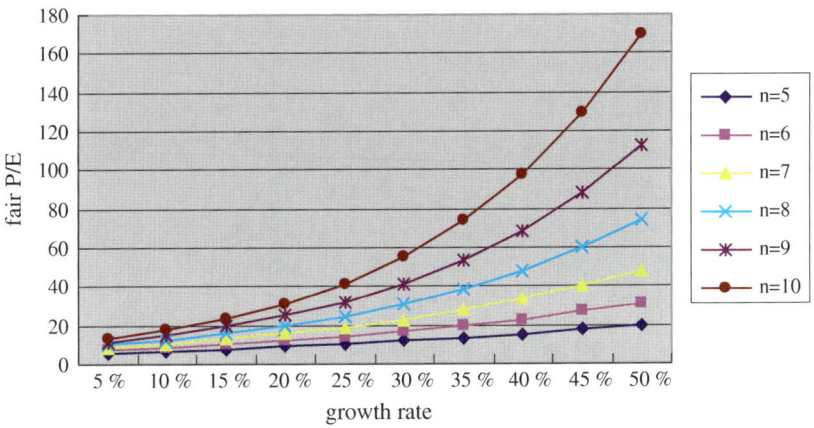

Fig. 3.5 Fair P/E curves based on the ZZ P/E model

the position of the FPC moves upward with the increasing of n. Hence, for relative valuation, if investors believe a stock will grow faster in the future, they should use a higher P/E to value it; similarly, if investors believe the stock will experience a dangerous future, they should use a shorter n or lower P/E to value it.

Some investors or analysts may be used to the "forward P/E", i.e. the ratio of the stock price to the earnings per share of next year. The original P/E can be converted easily into a "forward P/E". What we need to do is replacing E in Eq. 3.14 by $E/(1 + g)$, then:

$$P/E_{forward} = [(1+g)^n - 1]/g \qquad (3.15)$$

Comparing with Eqs. 3.14 and 3.15, when the growth rate is positive, which usually is the normal case, the original fair P/E is larger than the forward fair P/E. This is obviously in line with our intuition and real situation.

3.4.2 ZZ P/B Model

The P/B is the ratio of the stock price to the book value of its equity or net assets per share. Where, B is the net assets in the balance sheet divided by the firm's number of shares outstanding. As P/B ratio is also widely used in market and practical valuation, we now try to work out a fair or theoretical P/B model.

The earnings per share, E, is actually the product of the equity per share, B, and the return on equity (ROE). Let r to represent the ROE, then,

$$E = Br \qquad (3.16)$$

Therefore, the ZZ P/E model can be rewritten as:

$$P/E = P/(Br) = \left[(1+g)^n - 1\right](1+g)/g \qquad (3.17)$$

Hence,

$$P/B = \left[(1+g)^n - 1\right](1+g)r/g \qquad (3.18)$$

We referred to Eq. 3.18 as ZZ P/B model. Similarly, a new valuation model can be derived by rearranging the ZZ P/B model as:

$$P = \left[(1+g)^n - 1\right](1+g)Br/g \qquad (3.19)$$

Obviously, the theoretical P/B is the theoretical P/E multiplied by the return on equity. Similar to the ZZ P/E model, the data of independent variables in the ZZ P/B model are not difficult to estimate. It is worthy to mention that the return to equity r should be positive in valuation of a healthy firm or stock. In other words, it is the average return of the equity investment in normal situation in the future.

Comparing with the ZZ P/E model, the ZZ P/B model needs one more independent variable, r. Other things being equal, more variable means more estimated biases in the valuation. On the other hand, the value of an asset is strongly related to its future profitability and risk, while relative weakly related to its book value of net assets. Therefore, if both methods are feasible, the priority should be given to the ZZ P/E model.

Based on the ZZ P/B model (Eq. 3.18), Table 3.2 illustrates the theoretical P/Bs when the return on equity is assumed to be 20 %.

Table 3.2 The fair P/Bs when the return on equity is 20 %

n	g (%) −50	−40	−30	−20	−10	0	10	20
5	0.19	0.28	0.39	0.54	0.74	1.00	1.34	1.79
6	0.20	0.29	0.41	0.59	0.84	1.20	1.70	2.38
7	0.20	0.29	0.43	0.63	0.94	1.40	2.09	3.10
8	0.20	0.29	0.44	0.67	1.03	1.60	2.52	3.96
9	0.20	0.30	0.45	0.69	1.10	1.80	2.99	4.99
10	0.20	0.30	0.45	0.71	1.17	2.00	3.51	6.23

n	g (%) 30	40	50	60	70	80	90	100
5	2.35	3.06	3.96	5.06	6.41	8.05	10.03	12.40
6	3.32	4.57	6.23	8.41	11.24	14.86	19.44	25.20
7	4.57	6.68	9.65	13.78	19.45	27.10	37.32	50.80
8	6.20	9.63	14.78	22.37	33.40	49.14	71.29	102.0
9	8.32	13.76	22.47	36.12	57.11	88.81	135.8	204.4
10	11.08	19.55	34.00	58.11	97.43	160.2	258.4	409.2

3.4.3 ZZ P/S Model

It is easy to derive a ZZ P/S model via similar way as that of the ZZ P/B model. Let r' to be the profit margin, or the ratio of earnings (net income) to sales, earnings per share (E) equals sales per share (S) multiplied by the profit margin, i.e., E = Sr', then,

The ZZ P/E model can be rewritten as:

$$P/E = P/\left(Sr'\right) = \left[(1+g)^n - 1\right](1+g)/g \tag{3.20}$$

Hence,

$$P/S = \left[(1+g)^n - 1\right](1+g)r'/g \tag{3.21}$$

We referred to Eq. 3.21 as ZZ P/S model. Similarly, a valuation model can be derived by rearranging the ZZ P/S model:

$$P = \left[(1+g)^n - 1\right](1+g)Sr'/g \tag{3.22}$$

Obviously, the theoretical P/S is the theoretical P/E multiplied by the profit margin. The data of independent variables in the ZZ P/S model are not difficult to estimate or forecast. Similar with the ZZ P/B model, the profit margin r' should be positive in valuation of a healthy firm or stock. In other words, it is the "smoothed" profit margin of the firm in the future. Also, comparing with the ZZ P/E model, the ZZ P/S model needs one more independent variable. Therefore, to reduce the valuation biases, the priority should be given to the ZZ P/E model whenever it is feasible.

The P/S ratio has its advantages in valuation comparing with the P/E and P/B ratio. Some firms may experience a period of negative earnings, so it is hard to apply the P/E ratios to value their stocks; when these firms have relative less valuable or visible assets, or their actual values have weak links with their assets, the P/S will be the best ratio for valuation. In the reality, the P/S ratio is often used to value the high-tech or dot.com stocks, especially for the firms in their early stage when they have no stable positive earnings.

Based on the ZZ P/S model, Table 3.3 illustrates the theoretical P/Ss when the profit margin is assumed as 15 %.

In summary, we derive the theoretical P/E, P/B and P/S model based on the ZZ growth model; hence bridge the gap between the relative valuation and absolute valuation. The traditional experience-based P/E, P/B and P/S ratios are actually not convincing as a valuation benchmark, because the ratios of the market on average and the individual stocks are fluctuating endlessly and relative valuation itself cannot tell ratios on which day or average ratios over which period are the most correct. The theoretical P/E, P/B and P/S based on the ZZ growth model hence can play an irreplaceable role as the benchmarks in valuation, which is illustrated more clearly in the following section.

Table 3.3 The theoretical P/Ss when the profit margin is 15 %

n	g (%)							
	−50	−40	−30	−20	−10	0	10	20
5	0.15	0.21	0.29	0.40	0.55	0.75	1.01	1.34
6	0.15	0.21	0.31	0.44	0.63	0.90	1.27	1.79
7	0.15	0.22	0.32	0.47	0.70	1.05	1.57	2.32
8	0.15	0.22	0.33	0.50	0.77	1.20	1.89	2.97
9	0.15	0.22	0.34	0.52	0.83	1.35	2.24	3.74
10	0.15	0.22	0.34	0.54	0.88	1.50	2.63	4.67

n	g (%)							
	30	40	50	60	70	80	90	100
5	1.76	2.30	2.97	3.79	4.81	6.04	7.52	9.30
6	2.49	3.43	4.68	6.31	8.43	11.14	14.58	18.90
7	3.43	5.01	7.24	10.34	14.58	20.32	27.99	38.10
8	4.65	7.22	11.08	16.78	25.05	36.85	53.46	76.50
9	6.24	10.32	16.85	27.09	42.84	66.61	101.9	153.3
10	8.31	14.66	25.50	43.58	73.08	120.2	193.8	306.9

3.5 Some of the Applications of ZZ Growth Model and ZZ Ratio Models

Sound in theory, simple and feasible in practice, as a brand new absolute valuation approach, the ZZ growth model and ZZ ratio models have undoubtedly vast application potentials. The applications demonstrated in this section are by no means to prescribe some limits to the application of these models; rather, they are just some initial or rough examples for stimulating the use of these models.

3.5.1 Calculating the Fair-Priced Ratios

Value-based investments are recommended in market. Value-based investors should know first of all the values of the candidate stocks, or at least, know whether the candidate stocks as well as the market as a whole are over-valued or under-valued.

For instance, many countries have two stock markets: one is the market for traditional stocks, such as the New York Stock Exchange (NYSE), often referred to as main board in some countries; the other is for the high growth stocks, such as the Nasdaq (National Association of Securities Dealers Automated Quotations), often referred to as GEM (Growth Enterprises Market) board or the second board in some countries.

The ratios should vary across markets because stocks in different markets have different fundamentals concerning risk and return. While most investors know that

3.5 Some of the Applications of ZZ Growth Model and ZZ Ratio Models

the P/E, P/B and P/S of stocks in Nasdaq should be higher than that in NYSE, seldom among them know a method sound in theory for measuring the ratio differences, so that the investment decisions and regulation policies in reality have to be experience-oriented so far.

With the guidance of the theoretical ratios based on the ZZ ratios model, such as those shown in Tables 3.1, 3.2 and 3.3, the practical investment decision-making and regulation policy-making can be improved fundamentally.

For instance, if we believe that the growth rates of earnings on average are expected to be 10 % and 30 % over the future 10–20 years for the main board market and the second board market respectively; the required payback periods are 10 and 8 years for the investment in the main board market and in the second board market respectively, then the fair P/Es of the main board market and the second board market can be derived based on the ZZ P/E model:

$$P/E_{mainboard} = \left[(1 + 10\%)^{10} - 1\right](1 + 10\%)/10\% = 17.53$$

$$P/E_{secondboard} = \left[(1 + 30\%)^{8} - 1\right](1 + 30\%)/30\% = 31.01$$

As an investor, he/she can judge the deviation of the market from fair valuation based on the benchmark derived as above and decide his/her overall investment strategy, such as the mix of cash and stock positions. He/she can also judge the deviation of an individual stock from its fair value based on the benchmark derived from the ZZ P/E model and decide the investment strategy for that stock, such as the timing of buying and selling.

The regulators, such as who in the relevant government office and in the exchange, can announce the valuation benchmark of the market as a whole as well as the individual stocks derived from the ZZ P/E model as the guidance on some compulsory or voluntary bases to the market trading, so that reduce the manipulative and speculative behaviors in the market and keep the market more healthy and stable.

Although the theoretical P/E is not over sensible to the determinants of growth rate g and required payback period n, the two determinants themselves do have significant influences on the derived benchmark. The values of the two determinants will vary across persons to do the estimations, so the derived benchmarks based on a same correct financial model will be different for different persons.

This is not a problem worthy to worry about; rather, it is necessary for every stock to be traded on the market. Otherwise, as every one derives exactly a same fair value of a stock, the stock price will go fast toward this value, and then the trading volume of this stock will go down sharply to zero, because when every one believe the stock price equals its value, both the buying and selling of this stock are profitless and will be stopped in the market.

Anyway, the investors and regulators as well as the analysts themselves, are responsible to do their best to estimate the inputs. This is the general requirements for all the applications of financial models, just as what revealed in Chap. 1.

3.5.2 Measuring the Market Bubble

There are many important financial issues relied on the theoretical ratios. For instance, why has the measurement of market bubble been debated endlessly? The main reason is that no one has a theoretical ratio as a benchmark, whereas actual ratios cannot prove themselves are correct or incorrect. Once the theoretical P/E is known, it is easy to judge whether a market has bubble as well as whether a stock is over-valued.

Let us take China and the US Stock markets as the examples; and use the ZZ P/E model to measure the theoretical P/Es and the bubbles of the two markets.

The growth rate of GDP has been more or less than 10 % over past 20 years in China.[9] Considering the influence of the world wide financial crisis, assume all the listed firms in average will grow at 8 % annually over a foreseeable period in the future. Based on the average risk over the same period, suppose the investor required rate of return is 12.5 %, which implies the required payback period is 8 years. Then the fair or theoretical P/E is:

$$P/E = \left[(1+8\%)^8 - 1\right](1+8\%)/8\% = 11.49$$

Similarly, the growth rate of US GDP is around 5 % over past 20 years.[10] Considering the world wide financial crisis, assume the growth rate of all US listed firms is 4 % over a foreseeable period in the future, and the investor required payback period is also 8 years. Then the theoretical P/E is:

$$P/E = \left[(1+4\%)^8 - 1\right](1+4\%)/4\% = 9.58$$

The economic growth both in China and the U.S. can only support a theoretical P/E ratio around 10. The double growth rate of China can only support the P/E in China 1/5 ($\approx$11.49/9.58 $-$ 1) higher than that in the U.S. These secrets cannot be revealed by traditional financial research based on the historical data of P/Es or other ratios.

The fair or theoretical P/E is the bubble-free P/Es. As the bubble-free P/Es in China and in US market are about 11.49 and 9.58 respectively, the bubbles of the two markets cannot be easier to measure. If, for example, we find that one day, the actual P/Es are 20 and 15 in China and US market respectively, then the market bubble (MB):

$$MB_{China} = 20/11.49 - 1 = 74.06\%$$
$$MB_{US} = 15/9.58 - 1 = 56.58\%$$

---

[9] Based on data from Economic & Social Data Ranking (http://www.dataranking.com), GDP of China in 1985 and 2005 are 305.259 and 2,243.688 respectively. Thus average growth rate is 10.49 %.

[10] Based on data from Economic & Social Data Ranking (http://www.dataranking.com), GDP of the US in 1985 and 2005 are 4,220.250 and 12,455.825 respectively. Thus average growth rate is 5.56 %.

Therefore, when the theoretical P/E is known, the extent of the market bubble is easy to measure effectively and timely, which is the key to monitor and protect against financial crises. Thus, the model of the ZZ growth model and the ZZ ratio models solve two issues simultaneously: the valuation of stock and the measurement of market bubbles. As such, the appropriate applications of these models hopefully will enhance our ability greatly to guard against financial crises and stock market disasters.

3.5.3 Predicting the Change of Stock Price

Stock price fluctuates around its value. New findings or improvements on valuation thus benefit the predicting of stock price change. It is impossible to invent a model capable of predicting the change of stock price precisely, because the stock price goes around rather than equals its value for most of the time. It makes no sense to test a financial or valuation model based on the precision of stock price prediction in most cases.

As valuation models, the ZZ growth model and the ZZ ratio models can be used to predict stock price change associated with some events or policy. Although we cannot expect a precise prediction, the prediction can undoubtedly underpin the relevant investment decision-making and regulation policy-making.

Events and policies affecting stock prices via the value determinants, such as sales, cost, earnings, cash flows and the required rate of return of investors. So we can estimate the influences of the relevant events and policies on these value determinants; then apply the ZZ growth model and the ZZ ratio models to predict the appropriate stock price change.

Estimation of the change in stock value resulted from earnings change

Firms in reality can meet various events or changes during their operations. Such as fierce competition from other firms, the fluctuation of customers' demand (firms' sales), the change of cost especially the cost of inputs or the variable cost, the change of prevailing product price in the market, etc. These ever-changing conditions will influence the earnings of the relevant firms and their stock value and prices.

Consider that a firm runs into a sales change because of a change of production capability of the sector. According to the principle of the leverage of operating and financing, the change in sales will lead to a larger change in earnings. Suppose the relative change in the estimated earnings (decline or rise) is x over the foreseeable future. Use P and P' to represent the stock value before and after the sales and earnings change being forecasted respectively, based on the ZZ growth model:

$$P' = [(1+g)^n - 1](1+g) E (1+x)/g \qquad (3.23)$$

Based on Eq. 3.23 and Eq. 3.12, the relative change of the stock value X is:

$$X = P'/P - 1 = x \qquad (3.24)$$

The Eq. 3.24 implies the relative change of the stock value theoretically equals to the change of the earnings when the change of the earnings is expected to extend over and beyond the required payback period. Most sectors in reality experience a cycle or periodic change (up and down). So the earnings rise or decline may not remain over a long period. It thus makes sense to consider how long the change will last.

For example, a firm runs into a sales decline because new competitors move in. The estimated earnings decline is 30 % over the next 3 years; then earnings will recover to their original estimated levels (because some competitors move out) over the rest of the foreseeable period. Suppose the investors' required payback period (shorter than the foreseeable period) remains 8 years; the current earnings per share is 2 dollars; the original estimated annual average growth rate of the earnings is 15 %.

Stock value before the earnings change

$$P = [(1 + 15\%)^8 - 1](1 + 15\%) \times 2/15\% = 31.57$$

Stock value after the earnings change

$$P' = (1 - 30\%) \times 2 \times \sum_{t=1}^{3}(1 + 15\%)^{t+2} \times \sum_{t=4}^{8}(1 + 15\%)^t = 29.18$$

Hence, the relative change of the stock value X is:

$$X = 29.18/31.57 - 1 = -7.6\%$$

The decline of 7.6 % is much smaller than 30 %, which is the decline of the stock value based on Eq. 3.24 when the estimated earnings decline of 30 % will not be recovered over the foreseeable period. This reminds us that when we use the ZZ growth model and ZZ ratio models to predict the value or price change of a stock, be careful about the period assumption over which the influence of the relevant event will be lasting.

Obviously, the decline of the stock value should increase as the number of years before the earnings recover to the normal level increases. As for the above example, the special percentages of the decline in the stock value are shown in Table 3.4.

Estimation of the change in stock value resulted from interest change

In modern economy, the central bank often adjusts the national economy via the adjustment of interest rate. Both the investors and the central bank want to

Table 3.4 The decline of the stock value along with the number of years before the 30 % decline on earnings recover to the normal level

Number of years	1	2	3	4	5	6	7	8
Stock value	30.88	30.09	29.18	28.13	26.92	25.53	23.94	22.10
Value decline	−2.2 %	−4.7 %	−7.6 %	−10.9 %	−14.7 %	−19.1 %	−24.2 %	−30.0 %

3.5 Some of the Applications of ZZ Growth Model and ZZ Ratio Models

know how much the stock market will react to a certain interest rate adjustment. Let us analyze its influence on stock market based on the ZZ P/E model now.

Assume the central bank adjusts the interest rate scaled at x; the original investors' required rate of return is k. Other things (such as earnings) being equal, the investors' required rate of return after the interest adjustment should be k + x. Therefore, the required payback period of investors before and after the interest adjustment should be 1/k and 1/(k + x) respectively. Use P and P' to represent the stock price before and after the interest adjustment, based on the ZZ growth model:

$$P = \left[(1+g)^{1/k} - 1\right](1+g)E/g \tag{3.25}$$

$$P' = \left[(1+g)^{1/(k+x)} - 1\right](1+g)E/g \tag{3.26}$$

Hence, the relative change of the stock value X is

$$\begin{aligned}
X &= P'/P - 1 \\
&= \left\{\left[(1+g)^{1/(k+x)} - 1\right](1+g)E/g\right\} \Big/ \left\{\left[(1+g)^{1/k} - 1\right](1+g)E/g\right\} - 1 \\
&= \left[(1+g)^{1/(k+x)} - 1\right] \Big/ \left[(1+g)^{1/k} - 1\right] - 1
\end{aligned} \tag{3.27}$$

For example, consider stock H, the current earnings per share is 2 dollars; the estimated annual average growth rate of the earnings over foreseeable period (15 years or so) is 12 %; the original investors' required rate of return is 10 %; now the central bank cut down the interest rate by −0.5 %. Other things (such as earnings, etc.) being equal, the investors' required rate of return then should be 9.5 %. Based on Eq. 3.27:

$$X = \left[(1+12\%)^{1/9.5\%} - 1\right] \Big/ \left[(1+12\%)^{1/10\%} - 1\right] - 1 = 9.1\%$$

That is, other things being equal, the 0.5 % reduction in interest rate will result to a 9.1 % rise of the stock value or price. If there is no other important news in the market, once the interest rate reduction announced, investors can consider buying stock H when its price decline exceeds 9.1 %, or consider selling stock H when its price decline is less than 9.1 %.

The calculations about stock H can also be used to analyze the market as a whole. If the officers in the central bank want to smooth away the fluctuations of the stock market H with the fundamentals like the above stock H; and predict that the change of the various environmental factors will result to the stock prices go down about 9.1 %; then they can adopt a monetary policy to cut down the interest rate by 0.5 %.

The theoretical P/B and the theoretical P/S are also bubble-free ratios, hence can also be used to calculate the fair ratios, to measure the bubbles of market and the specific stocks and to predict the change of stock price associated with some events, just like the applications of the ZZ P/E model and the ZZ growth model. As the processes are similar and easy, we do not intend to illustrate their applications one by one further.

3.6 Summary

The series of valuation models in this chapter, i.e. the theoretical P/E, P/B and P/S models as well as the ZZ growth models represent a brand new way in valuation and an innovation in finance. These models solve the key valuation issues in absolute valuation—avoid the ZZ growth paradox trouble by replacing the required rate of return with the required payback period as the criterion; the valuation models are flexible enough to value individual stock across sectors and the growth rate as a key input is feasible to be forecasted. These models solve as well the key valuation issues in relative valuation—provide an effective way to find the theoretical ratios in valuation as well as to measure the bubbles of the individual stocks and the overall market. Consequently, these models bridge the gap between the relative valuation and the absolute valuation. These features betoken the vast potentials in theory and practice of this brand new valuation approach.

References

1. Gordon MJ (1962) The savings investment and valuation of a corporation. Rev Econ Stat 44(1):37–51
2. Damodaran A (2006) Damodaran on valuation: security analysis for investment and corporate finance. John Wiley & Sons, Inc
3. Black F, Scholes M (1973) The pricing of options and corporate liabilities. J Polit Econ 81(3):637–654
4. Merton R (1973) Theory of rational option pricing. Bell J Econ Manage Sci 4(1):141–183
5. Cox JC, Ross SA, Rubinstein M (1979) Option pricing: a simplified approach. J Financ Econ 7:229–263
6. Hull JC (2012) Options, Futures, and Other Derivatives, 8th edn. Pearson Education Limited.

Chapter 4
Certainty Equivalent, Risk Premium and Asset Pricing

We reveal in Chap. 2 that finance as a science is just on its initial stage; we even cannot make sure whether the very long term growth rate of asset returns is positive or negative. In front of the ZZ growth paradox, the widely used Gordon growth model is actually invalid (just something for show). We solve the problem with a brand new valuation method under the criterion of required payback period in Chap. 3.

Anyway, if we do not adopt a perpetual (or very long term) growth rate as a variable in the model, the DCF method may make some sense, such as that in capital budgeting or project evaluation. The application of DCF method needs necessarily a discount rate, which is determined conceptually by the investors' required rate of return, which is further determined theoretically by the asset risk. The discount rate hence can be referred to as risk-adjusted discount rate or the investors' required rate of return. While we focus mainly on the return side in last chapter, we now turn on to the risk side in this chapter.

Apart from the asset returns, the investors' required return or risk-adjusted discount rate, k, as another key input for DCF method, is also lack of plausible methods to estimate. Obviously, if we cannot determine a convincing discount rate in theory, most (if not all) valuation and financial analyses make no sense. This is the intention of this chapter.

4.1 Alternatives to Determine a Discount Rate

All financial analyses and decisions, including investment, financing, risk assessment, valuation and so on, should be based on the future cash flows. Those predicted or estimated future cash flows are their expected values; their actual possible values are supposed to lie around the expected values and often following a normal distribution. Therefore, such predicted or expected values contain uncertainty or risk.

Financial decisions rely on the trade-off between risk and return. It is important to incorporate the risk well into the decisions. As the DCF method becomes the basic or even the only approach for valuation and finance analyses, analysts are used to consider risk via the discount rate. As indicated in Chap. 1, the basic indicator of risk is the standard deviation or variance of asset returns. For considering risk via discount rate, an effective method is necessary to determine: when the standard deviation or variance increases by, say 1 %, how much should the discount rate change?

There are multiple alternatives to determine the discount rate in finance-related textbooks and in practice. Unfortunately, none of them can answer the above simple question. We now examine them one by one.

4.1.1 The Industrial Average Rate of Return

Some financial and investment textbooks take the industrial average rate of return as a benchmark to determine the discount rate. This may have some advantage in data availability, but may be far from reaching a correct decision. Although high returns are often associated with high risks; it is by no means that the returns in a specific industry over a past specific period represent the appropriate risk premium in future.

In fact, in any given industry and geographic area at any given time, the market is likely to be inefficient for various reasons; the risks in some industries may be over compensated by the average returns; whereas the risks in other industries may be under compensated by the average returns. This is the very reason for industries to be different in attractiveness, and also the primary motivation for capitals to transfer across industries.

For instance, a firm needs to choose one between two exclusive projects. Project A is in the traditional industry that the firm is currently operating in; project B is in a high growth industry. The current average returns of the traditional industry and high growth industry are 5 % and 30 % respectively. The estimated returns on project A and B are 6 % and 28 % respectively. If the firm uses 5 % and 30 % as the discount rate respectively for project A and B, the decision is accepting A and rejecting B. Is this a right choice?

General speaking, accepting A and rejecting B implies that the firm chooses a 6 % return at the cost of a 28 % return. This seems a bad choice. If the risk in the high growth industry is not significantly higher than the traditional industry, accepting A and rejecting B is definitely a wrong decision. Obviously, to make a right choice, the firm needs compare the returns of 6 % and 28 % with the risk-matched (i.e. risk adjusted) discount rates rather than the average rate of returns respectively in the two industries.

4.1.2 The Opportunity Cost of Capital

The opportunity cost of capital is widely adopted as the discount rate without any attention on the uncertainty of the opportunity cost itself.

4.1 Alternatives to Determine a Discount Rate

As a concept from economics, opportunity cost is created for decision-making. Economics tells us that we need to choose because of the scarcity of resources (such as assets). When we make a choice (i.e. make a decision), we forgo other alternatives to use the asset. The opportunity cost is the return of the best one among all the forgone alternatives. Therefore, if the opportunity cost lower than the return of the chosen alternative, the decision (choice) is right; otherwise, the decision (choice) is wrong.

Believe it or not, the opportunity cost illustrates perfectly the important features of economics (as indicated in Chap. 1): decision-oriented but not necessarily feasible. For most resources, such as capitals, there are numerous alternatives to use (invest). While choosing the best alternative within a limited range is not difficult, making the best choice among all forgone alternatives is too difficult to accomplish, because there are numerous forgone alternatives to invest the capitals in terms of the nations, areas, industries, sectors, projects, sizes, technologies, models, assets, partners as well as the mixes of these factors.

In fact, opportunity cost may be more useful for explanation after the decision rather than for decision-making in advance. As for determining the opportunity cost of capital, different analysts or decision makers have different views about the potential opportunities for the capital; hence will inevitably work out different opportunity costs of a certain capital. In such a way, which opportunity cost of capital is right to be the discount rate? A question is: why do we determine the discount rate based especially on the returns of other forgone projects which is nothing to do with the risk of the invested project?

Therefore, it is neither feasible nor reasonable to determine the discount rate based on the opportunity cost of the capital.

4.1.3 The Weighted Average Cost of Capital

Most (if not all) financial, investment and valuation books as well as related research papers confuse the cost of capital and the discount rate and often adopt the weighted average cost of capital (WACC) as the discount rate for valuing assets and projects. Actually, capital cost and discount rate are different from each other. Capital cost is the result of financing (decision), and may have nothing to do with the asset risk. Asset or its risk is the result of investment (decision), and definitely has much to do with the discount rate.

The reason to discount the future cash flows is that investors need two compensations: one is the compensation for the deferment of returns, which can be referred to as time premium; the other is the compensation for the risk of returns, which can be referred to as risk premium. Therefore, the discount rate should be the sum of the time premium and the risk premium. As future cash flows are definitely later in time and have some uncertainties, both the time premium and the risk premium are positive. Hence the discount rate is definitely positive, or cannot be zero or negative in theory.

On the contrary, the capital cost, no matter equity capital or debt capital, can be negative in theory, although it is not common in reality. Consider a corporate bond with face value 1000 dollars, coupon rate 10 %, and 8 years to maturity. How much is the capital cost of this bond if its issuing price is 1900 dollars? Although it is unusual for a bond with these features to issue at a price over 1800 dollars, if there is a unusual reason that the proceeds is indeed more than 1800 dollars for every bond issued, obviously, the capital cost of this bond can only be negative in such a case. It is more possible for an equity or stock (than for a bond or a debt) to issue at an over high price, which implies the capital cost of equity may be more likely to be negative.

Most finance-related books and research papers state that the cost of equity is higher than the cost of debt. This is a similar mistake resulted from the concept chaos about capital cost and discount rate. As the result of financing, equity cost is not necessarily higher than debt cost. There are multiple factors influencing the issuing prices of both equity and debt. When the equity is issuing at a very high price, its cost is obviously possible to be lower than the debt cost or even can be negative. This is the primary reason for listed firms in China to prefer equity financing rather than debt financing. Thus, capital cost depends on the related financing decisions, or the securities issuing prices.

Therefore, the cost of capital can be positive or negative, whereas the discount rate can only be positive; the discount rate for equity investment should be higher than that for debt investment; whereas the equity cost can be higher or lower than the debt cost depending on the issuing price of the relevant equity and debt. Thus, after revising the confused concepts about the capital cost and discount rate, it is clear that capital cost has nothing to do with the asset risk; it is not theoretically sound to determine the discount rate based on capital cost; no matter it is opportunity cost, equity cost or weighted average cost.

Although finance is still on its initial stage, it is beneficial for both investment decision and financing decision by distinguishing capital cost and discount rate. On one hand, financing decision is also an important and independent decision in most firms. Other things being equal, good financing decisions will lower firms' capital costs. The capital cost hence is an important indicator for firms to evaluate their financing decisions. Otherwise, if a financing decision is evaluated based on the discount rate, the evaluation makes no sense because the discount rate has nothing to do with the efforts in financing decision.

On the other hand, misusing capital cost as discount rate may lead to mistakes in investment decision. For instance, firm A and firm B are seeking good projects. They find project X and have the same views on the risk and return of it. The annual estimated returns of project X is 30 % for both A and B. However, the capital cost is 10 % in firm A, and is 30 % in firm B as a result of some financing mistakes. Now, how can A and B make their decisions on project X? If they misuse their capital cost as the discount rate (guided by the prevailing textbooks), A will accept X; and B will reject X.

Unfortunately, this is not right to make the decision, because there is no chance that A and B are both correct this way. Just think what will happen after that?

After that, A will invest in X and operate; B will go on to seek better projects. There are obviously two possibilities. One is that B succeeds to find a better project. If it is true, the decision of A is wrong. The second possibility is that B fails to find a better project. If it is true, the decision of B is wrong; because during the period in which A runs X and gets annual returns of 30 %, B can only gets a much lower returns on its unused capital (for instance just deposit the capital in bank and gets the poor interest) although the cost of this capital is 30 %. Obviously, the logic dilemma is coming from the wrong choice of the discount rate.

Actually, capital cost as the result of financing is irrelevant to investment decision. It is wrong to incorporate irrelevant cost into consideration for decision-makings.

4.1.4 The Capital Asset Pricing Model

None of the above alternatives in determining discount rate is right in theory, though they are widely used in practice and widely spread in textbooks. As such, it is urgent to find a convincing method or model to determine the discount rate, because valuation is the core function of finance and the discount rate is an inevitable input for the prevailing valuation. Obviously, a theoretically correct method or model is needed to determine the discount rate based on the risk of the project or asset under consideration. The method or model should be able to answer the question like: when the standard deviation or variance of the asset's expected returns increases by, say 1 %, how much should the discount rate change?

About 50 years ago, William Sharpe finds a model to describe the theoretical or fair relationship between return and risk.[1] Such a model, if it is correct in theory, can be used to determine the investors' required rate of return or risk adjusted discount rate based on the asset risk. Sharpe's model takes the form:

$$E(R_i) = R_f + \beta_i [E(R_m) - R_f] \quad (4.1)$$

where:

$E(R_i)$ is the expected or required rate of return on the ith capital asset;
R_f is the risk free interest rate such as the yield to maturity of a government bond;
β_i (the beta coefficient) is the sensitivity of the asset returns to market returns;
$E(R_m)$ is the expected rate of return of the market;
$E(R_m) - R_f$ is known as the average market risk premium.

Sharpe's model is referred to as capital asset pricing model (CAPM). The CAPM states that the appropriate rate of return on an asset is the sum of a risk free rate and a risk premium. The risk free rate represents the compensation to

---

[1] See Ref. [1]. John Lintner (1962) and Jan Mossin (1966) also introduced the model independently; Sharpe finds the CAPM around the end of 1962 and publishes it in 1964.

the deferment of the return; and the risk premium represents the compensation to the risk of the investment (to the asset). It seems that the structure of return in the CAPM is reasonable and correct.

Further, the risk premium in CAPM is the product of two factors. One is the average risk premium of the market, i.e. $E(R_m) - R_f$; the second is the Beta coefficient of the asset, i.e. β_i. As the market risk premium is given, the Beta coefficient (or simply referred to as Beta) measures the asset risk. Hence Beta has been a new risk indicator since Sharpe's CAPM.

Sharpe's CAPM is the first strict model to describe the relationship between risk and return. It is actually the only theoretical model so far.[2] Apart from Sharpe's CAPM, no model describes clearly and certainly about the risk-return relationship. Hence this model is widely used in determining the appropriate discount rate. William Sharpe wins his Nobel Prize in Economics in 1990 for his remarkable contribution in finance.

However, for the risk considerations, Sharpe's CAPM takes into account only the systematic risk or market risk rather than the total risk or the firm (or project) risk. In other words, the risk premium determined by Sharpe's CAPM is only systematic risk premium on the assumption that the nonsystematic risk is completely canceled out by diversified investment. This is obviously not in line with the reality. In most situations when a firm makes financial decisions (such as investment decision), it should take into account both the systematic risk and the non-systematic risk. Therefore Sharpe's CAPM is actually not enough for incorporating the relevant risk in financial decisions.

Therefore, Sharpe's CAPM is actually cannot save financial theory from the crisis resulted from the discount rate determination, although financial community blinds to this crisis with a fragile excuse that all nonsystematic risk can be canceled out.

4.2 Certainty Equivalent and Risk Equivalent

It is just one way to consider risk via discount rate in valuation and finance; another way is to consider risk via the returns (cash flows or earnings) being discounted. Specifically speaking, if we can transform the predicted returns being discounted into their certainty equivalents, which are smaller than their original predicted returns because of the risks, we then need to discount the certainty equivalents only at risk free rate. In other words, the certainty equivalents in future need only time compensations.

We now try to do this.

---

[2] Arbitrage pricing theory (APT) initiated by Stephen Ross in 1976 also describes the return and risk relation. APT holds that the expected return of an asset can be modeled as a linear function of various macro-economic factors or theoretical market indices, where sensitivity to changes in each factor is represented by a factor-specific beta coefficient. However, as a model based on empirical data, the APT has no certain variables and model form, thus it is not theoretical sound and it is less popular in academic and practical research.

4.2.1 On Certainty Equivalent

The "certainty equivalent" is a good suggestion to incorporate risk in valuation and financial decisions. Traditionally, the certainty equivalent is defined as a certain return as equally attractive to investors as the corresponding predicted or expected uncertain return.

However, neither academic nor practical efforts so far can provide a convenient and reliable method to work out this certainty equivalent. In practice as well as in many textbooks, the suggested method to obtain the certainty equivalent is the experience-based subjective estimation. Specifically, in order to transfer the predicted value of return into its "certainty equivalent", one should determine first a "certainty equivalent coefficient" (referred to as certainty coefficient hereafter) based on "experience"; then multiply the predicted return by the "certainty coefficient" to get the certainty equivalent of the return.

Understandingly, the certainty coefficient varies between 0 and 1, because the certainty equivalent is smaller than its corresponding predicted or expected value, and it increases as the estimated risk decreases. These are all we know so far about the certainty equivalent and the certainty coefficient. Beyond such basic knowledge, like what are the common influential factors, what are the relations between the certainty coefficient and its influential variables, and so on, are all unknown. Many people even believe that the influential factors of the certainty coefficient vary too much across cases and firms, it is impossible to abstract common key variables and build a general model.

Although the concept of the certainty equivalent is constructive, it cannot play a proper role in finance and valuation without an effective model. In addition, as there is no effective method to determine the risk premium, most of the financial calculations are lack of theoretical foundation without the reliable certainty equivalents. Take NPV (net present value) as an example. Being widely regarded as the most perfect method in capital budgeting, if only the systematic risk rather than the total risk can be incorporated in the evaluation, the NPV method is actually just something for show.

There are indeed some (but not many) scholars try to model the certainty equivalent, such as Gordon [2], Becker and Sarin [3], Kimball (1993), Gollier and Pratt [4], Rabin [5], Hennessy and Lapan [6], etc. However, these studies stem from an identical idea: the certainty equivalent of an uncertain future value is the certain value that can bring in the same expected utility without risk. Therefore, the problem of modeling the equivalent is translated into the problem of modeling the utility. These studies thus rely completely on the utility function. Unfortunately, the utility, as an economic concept, is neither objective nor measurable; there is no possibility to build an objective or reliable model of utility.

Seems no way out? Again, do not give up! This chapter will provide efficient solutions for modeling the certainty equivalent as well as other alternatives to incorporating total risk into valuations and financial decisions.

4.2.2 Risk Equivalent Model

The certainty equivalent is smaller than its corresponding expected value. We define the difference between the expected value and the certainty equivalent as the risk equivalent. Use X to represent the predicted or expected value, d to represent the certainty coefficient, CE to represent the certainty equivalent and RE to represent the risk equivalent, then

$$RE = X - CE \tag{4.2}$$

$$CE = X - RE = Xd \tag{4.3}$$

Equation 4.3 transfers the problem of modeling the certainty equivalent into the problem of modeling the risk equivalent, i.e. the certainty equivalent is its corresponding expected value minus the value reduction caused by the risk. Therefore, the next step is naturally to scrutinize and value the risk. As a general definition, risk is uncertainty. According to the common sense, risk here is mainly refers to the situation that the actual value of a return is lower than its predicted value.

As shown in Fig. 4.1, S represents the possible values of the predicted return; X represents the special predicted value of the return in year T. Obviously, every point on a straight line x embarking from the zero point and upright rising at 45° always has a scale at the ordinate (vertical) axis equaling its scale at the abscissa (horizontal) axis. Suppose point E on this line is the predicted point with scales at both axes being X. Therefore, the risk is represented by the line segment OE, which is part of the line x below the point E.

In order to eliminate such risk, i.e. to keep the actual point not dropping down along the line x below E when S is smaller than X, we need a guarantee. The guarantee functions (provides value) as the dashed line shown in Fig. 4.1, which is obviously a put option. Comparing with the risk free situation, the predicted value

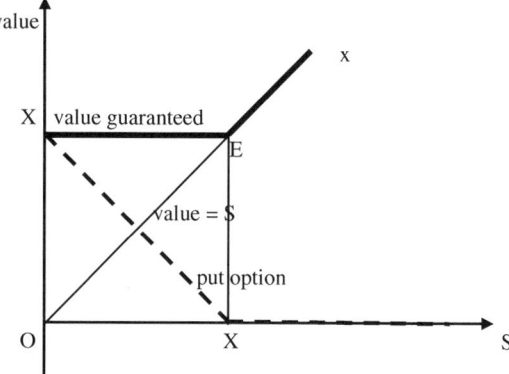

Fig. 4.1 risk equivalent = guarantee = put option

4.2 Certainty Equivalent and Risk Equivalent

needs a guarantee or a put. This implies that the risk equivalent equals the value of the put.

Therefore, we can find the risk equivalent by valuing the put. According to Fig. 4.1, the guarantee is to guarantee the value not lower than the X at the due time. It thus is a standard European put option. The most convenient way to value such a put is using the Black–Scholes option pricing model, as introduced in last chapter:

$$p = Xe^{-rT}N(-d2) - SN(-d1) \tag{4.4}$$

where, S is the current value of the underlying asset; X is the strike price of the put; T is the option maturity time; r is the risk-free discount rate, which can be determined based on the short-term government bonds. N(−d2) and N(−d1) represent the cumulative probability under standard normal distribution when the variable equals −d2 and −d1 respectively, and d1 and d2 can be derived with the following equations:

$$d1 = \frac{\ln(S/X) + (r + \sigma^2/2)T}{\sigma\sqrt{T}} \tag{4.5}$$

$$d2 = \frac{\ln(S/X) + (r - \sigma^2/2)T}{\sigma\sqrt{T}} = d1 - \sigma\sqrt{T} \tag{4.6}$$

where σ is the annual standard deviation of the return on the underlying asset, often called as the (underlying) asset volatility.[3] Note that the numerator of Eq. 4.5, $\ln(S/X) + (r + \sigma^2/2)T = \ln(S/X) + rT + \sigma^2T/2 = \ln(S/X) + \ln(e^{rT}) + \sigma^2T/2 = \ln[S/(Xe^{-rT})] + \sigma^2T/2$. Similarly, the numerator of Eq. 4.6, $\ln(S/X) + (r - \sigma^2/2)T = \ln[S/(Xe^{-rT})] - \sigma^2T/2$. For the convenience of application, I would like to transform the Eqs. 4.5 and 4.6 as:

$$d1 = \frac{\ln[S/(Xe^{-rT})]}{\sigma\sqrt{T}} + \frac{\sigma\sqrt{T}}{2} \tag{4.7}$$

$$d2 = \frac{\ln[S/(Xe^{-rT})]}{\sigma\sqrt{T}} - \frac{\sigma\sqrt{T}}{2} = d1 - \sigma\sqrt{T} \tag{4.8}$$

As for our analysis of risk equivalent, in Eqs. 4.4, 4.7 and 4.8, S is the current value of the predicted value; X is the predicted value at the maturity date; T is the

---

[3] According to prior empirical research, the volatilities of stock returns in traditional industries usually range from 20 % to 60 %, such as Turner and Weigel [7], etc. Thus, if the sector or the firm is relative riskier, then the volatility is closer to 60 %; if the sector or the firm is relative safer, then the volatility is closer to 20 %.

maturity time at which the return X will occur; σ is the annual standard deviation of the relative change of the predicted value; r is the risk free rate. In a risk neutral environment as assumed in option pricing model, various values of outlays and returns grow or discount at the risk free interest rate in the way of continuous compounding.

The put or the guarantee is to guarantee the predicted value not less than X at time T. Therefore, the X and T here are identical as that in the Black–Scholes option pricing model. In a risk neutral environment, S is the present value of the relevant variable which is expected to be X in time T. Then the $S = Xe^{-rT}$. Therefore, $\ln[S/(Xe^{-rT})] = \ln[(Xe^{-rT})/(Xe^{-rT})] = 0$. According to Eqs. 4.7 and 4.8, for valuing the risk equivalent:

$$d1 = \frac{\ln[S/(Xe^{-rT})]}{\sigma\sqrt{T}} + \frac{\sigma\sqrt{T}}{2} = \frac{\sigma\sqrt{T}}{2} = \sigma\sqrt{T/4} \quad (4.9)$$

$$d2 = \frac{\ln[S/(Xe^{-rT})]}{\sigma\sqrt{T}} - \frac{\sigma\sqrt{T}}{2} = -\frac{\sigma\sqrt{T}}{2} = -\sigma\sqrt{T/4} \quad (4.10)$$

Hence,

$$P = Xe^{-rT}N(-d2) - SN(-d1)$$
$$= Xe^{-rT}[N(-d2) - N(-d1)]$$
$$= Xe^{-rT}[N(\sigma\sqrt{T/4}) - N(-\sigma\sqrt{T/4})]$$
$$= Xe^{-rT}\{N(\sigma\sqrt{T/4}) - [1 - N(\sigma\sqrt{T/4})]\}$$

Or,

$$P = Xe^{-rT}[2N(\sigma\sqrt{T/4}) - 1] \quad (4.11)$$

Note that the certainty equivalent and the risk equivalent as well as the corresponding predicted or expected value are all occurring at the due time T, rather than occurring at present. However, the value of the put derived from the Black–Scholes model is a present value. Therefore, we should bring the above put value back to its "future value" for the purpose of valuing the risk equivalent, i.e.,

$$RE = Pe^{rT}$$
$$= Xe^{-rT}[2N(\sigma\sqrt{T/4}) - 1]e^{rT} \quad (4.12)$$
$$= X[2N(\sigma\sqrt{T/4}) - 1]$$

Equation 4.12 is the model of risk equivalent.

4.2 Certainty Equivalent and Risk Equivalent

4.2.3 Certainty Equivalent Model

Based on Eqs. 4.3 and 4.12,

$$\begin{aligned} CE &= X - RE \\ &= X - X[2N(\sigma\sqrt{T/4}) - 1] \\ &= 2X[1 - N(\sigma\sqrt{T/4})] \end{aligned} \quad (4.13)$$

Equation 4.13 is the model of certainty equivalent.
Further, based on Eqs. 4.3 and 4.13,

$$d = CE/X = 2[1 - N(\sigma\sqrt{T/4})] \quad (4.14)$$

Equation 4.14 is the model of certainty coefficient. Corresponding to the certainty coefficient, we define and model the risk equivalent coefficient, or risk coefficient, v:

$$v = 1 - d = 2N(\sigma\sqrt{T/4}) - 1 \quad (4.15)$$

Based on Eqs. 4.14 and 4.15, the certainty coefficient and the risk coefficient depend on two factors, i.e. two common influential factors: the volatility σ and the time horizon T. So we finally abstract the common influential factors of certainty equivalent, risk equivalent and their coefficients. As a common sense, increase in the volatility σ and the time horizon T will decrease the certainty coefficient and increase the risk coefficient. At one extreme, when one of the volatility σ and the time horizon T approaches infinite value, the certainty coefficient will be zero and the risk coefficient will be 1; At another extreme, when one of the volatility σ and the time horizon T approaches zero, the certainty coefficient will be 1 and the risk coefficient will be zero.

Let us examine the outcomes of the Eqs. 4.14 and 4.15. When the σ or T equals 0, $\sigma\sqrt{T/4} = 0$, $N(\sigma\sqrt{T/4}) = 0.5$, $d = 1$ and $v = 0$; when the σ or T approaches ∞, $\sigma\sqrt{T/4} = \infty$, $N(\sigma\sqrt{T/4}) = 1$, $d = 0$ and $v = 1$. Thus, these models illustrate that: the certainty coefficient reaches its maximum of 1 and the risk coefficient reaches its minimum of 0 for today's or certain "predicted" value; the certainty coefficient reaches its minimum of 0 and the risk coefficient reaches its maximum of 1 for the infinite future or completely uncertain "predicted" value; the larger of the volatility or/and the further of the time distance, the bigger of the risk equivalent and the smaller of the certainty equivalent.

These features obviously make sense and imply that the certainty coefficient model and the risk coefficient model (Eqs. 4.14 and 4.15) as well as the risk equivalent model and the certainty equivalent model (Eqs. 4.12 and 4.13) are correct in theory. To distinguish conveniently from other certainty equivalent related models (such as those based on utility functions), I refer to the Eqs. 4.12–4.15 as ZZ risk equivalent model (ZZ RE model), ZZ certainty equivalent model (ZZ CE model), ZZ certainty equivalent coefficient model (ZZ CEC model), ZZ risk equivalent coefficient model (ZZ REC model) respectively.

4.2.4 Exemplifications

As a fundamental innovation in finance, the ZZ certainty equivalent related models can be used in various financial analyses and decisions, especially when we have no effective model to incorporate total risk into valuation and financial decisions. We illustrate in this section some basic applications of this series of models in capital budgeting and risk pricing based on a simple numerical example.

Consider a project G, the initial capital outlay and the predicted follow-up cash flows each year during the 10 years' project life are shown in Table 4.1. In addition, the annual risk free rate is 5 % which assumed to be unchanged in 10 years.

4.2.4.1 NPV Calculation

If we do not care the risk at all, we can use the risk free rate 5 % to discount the predicted cash flows. Under such circumstances, the NPV of this project is:

$$\text{NPV} = \sum_{t=1}^{10} \frac{CF_t}{(1+5\,\%)^t} - CF_0$$
$$= 384.26 - 200 = 184.26$$

Now, assume the firm will consider risk via the certainty equivalent. If the firm believes the appropriate volatility is 25 %, based on the ZZ CE model and the ZZ CEC model, the certainty coefficient and the certainty equivalent are shown in Table 4.2.

Table 4.1 Cash flows forecasted for project G

years	0	1	2	3	4	5	6	7	8	9	10
Cash flow	−200	10	30	50	70	90	90	70	50	30	10

Table 4.2 The certainty equivalents of the predicted cash flows (volatility is 25 %)

Years	0	1	2	3	4	5	6	7	8	9	10
Cash flow	−200	10	30	50	70	90	90	70	50	30	10
CEC	1.00	0.90	0.86	0.83	0.80	0.78	0.76	0.74	0.72	0.71	0.69
CE	−200	9.01	25.79	41.43	56.18	70.19	68.35	51.86	36.18	21.23	6.93

CEC certainty coefficient, *CE* certainty equivalent

4.2 Certainty Equivalent and Risk Equivalent

Table 4.3 The certainty equivalents of the predicted cash flows (volatility is 15 %)

Years	0	1	2	3	4	5	6	7	8	9	10
Cash flow	−200	10	30	50	70	90	90	70	50	30	10
CEC	1.00	0.94	0.92	0.90	0.88	0.87	0.85	0.84	0.83	0.82	0.81
CE	−200	9.40	27.47	44.83	61.65	78.01	76.88	58.99	41.60	24.66	8.13

CEC certainty coefficient, *CE* certainty equivalent

Theoretically, the certainty equivalent should be discounted at risk free rate. Discounting the certainty equivalents in Table 4.2 at 5 %, the NPV of the project G is:

$$\text{NPV} = \sum_{t=1}^{10} \frac{CE_t}{(1+5\%)^t} - CE_0$$
$$= 299.26 - 200 = 99.26$$

If the firm believes the appropriate volatility is 15 % rather than 25 %, then the certainty coefficient and the certainty equivalent are shown in Table 4.3.

Discounting the certainty equivalents in Table 4.3 at 5 %, the NPV of the project G is,

$$\text{NPV} = \sum_{t=1}^{10} \frac{CE_t}{(1+5\%)^t} - CE_0$$
$$= 332.78 - 200 = 132.78$$

In the above calculations and in Tables 4.2 and 4.3, the certainty coefficient decreases as the "maturity", T, and the volatility, σ, increase. These are the insights we get from the ZZ certainty coefficient model and ZZ risk coefficient model beyond the traditional common knowledge that certainty coefficient ranges from 0 to 1.

4.2.4.2 Risk Pricing

In addition to incorporate the risk in investment decision, the certainty coefficient and risk coefficient models, of course, can be used to support other related decisions. For instance, in reality, there are indeed guarantees or insurances for promising corresponding cash flows or values, these kinds of guarantees or insurances may be priced based on the certainty coefficient and the risk coefficient. Tables 4.4 and 4.5 calculate the risk coefficient and the risk equivalent of the corresponding cash flows in Tables 4.2 and 4.3.

Table 4.4 The risk equivalent of the predicted cash flow (volatility is 25 %)

Years	0	1	2	3	4	5	6	7	8	9	10
Cash flow	−200	10	30	50	70	90	90	70	50	30	10
REC	0.00	0.10	0.14	0.17	0.20	0.22	0.24	0.26	0.28	0.29	0.31
RE	0.00	0.99	4.21	8.57	13.82	19.81	21.65	18.14	13.82	8.77	3.07

REC risk equivalent coefficient, *RE* risk equivalent

Table 4.5 The risk equivalent of the predicted cash flow (volatility is 15 %)

Years	0	1	2	3	4	5	6	7	8	9	10
Cash flow	−200	10	30	50	70	90	90	70	50	30	10
REC	0.00	0.06	0.08	0.10	0.12	0.13	0.15	0.16	0.17	0.18	0.19
RE	0.00	0.60	2.53	5.17	8.35	11.99	13.12	11.01	8.40	5.34	1.87

REC risk equivalent coefficient, *RE* risk equivalent

For consistency, we use the same discount rate to discount the predicted value, the certainty equivalent and the risk equivalent. Based on the volatility 25 %, the sum of the present value of each year's risk equivalent is 85.00, which is just the difference between the total value of the project without consideration of risk and the total present value of its certainty equivalent, i.e. $384.26 - 299.26 = 85.00$. Obviously, ignoring the transaction cost (such as the operating cost and profit of the guarantee or the insurance company), the fair price of the guarantee or the insurance for the predicted cash flows should be 85.00.

Based on the volatility 15 %, the sum of the present value of each year's risk equivalent is 51.48, which is also just the difference between the total value of the project without consideration of risk and the total value of its certainty equivalent, i.e. $384.26 - 332.78 = 51.48$. Similarly, neglecting the transaction cost, the fair price of the guarantee or the insurance for the predicted cash flows should be 51.48. This fair price is lower than that when the volatility is 25 % (85.00), which obviously makes sense.

When it is hard to estimate the variable σ, to follow the conservative principle in decision making, the guarantee or insurance company can somewhat overestimate it, hence derive a relative high risk value. However, to compete efficiently, it is obviously very important to estimate the σ and to calculate the risk coefficient hence the risk value as precisely as possible. On the other hand, it is also important to know the value of the guarantee or the insurance for the guaranteed or the insured firms.

The discovery of new and effective pricing method may be possible to play roles beyond what illustrated in the above example, i.e., set a standard or guidance for pricing. Pricing is an essential step for financial innovation. For the guarantee or insurance firms or other financial firms, new and more effective pricing method may be a must for their business expansion. For instance, the celebrated Black–Scholes model and its applications have been a key ingredient to the booming of various financial derivatives in past decades.

4.3 Risk Premium and a New CAPM

4.3.1 Modeling Risk Premium and a New CAPM

As mentioned previously, the reasons to discount include time compensation (time premium) and risk compensation (risk premium). The discount rate is the sum of the time premium and the risk premium, just as what demonstrated in Sharpe's CAPM.

4.3 Risk Premium and a New CAPM

The common financial calculation "discounting" hence can be divided into two steps: (1) risk discounting—discount the risky or uncertain cash flow at risk premium to get its certainty equivalent at due time; (2) time discounting—discount the certainty equivalent at risk free rate (time premium) to get its value at present time.

This implies the certainty equivalent conceptually is the result of discounting the expected value at the risk premium. Therefore, the certainty coefficient can be regarded as the "risk discount factor". Correspondingly, 1 discounting at the risk free rate is the "time discount factor". Use c to denote the annual risk premium and assume discounting the risk in the same way of "continuous-compounding discounting", then

$$d = 2[1 - N(\sigma\sqrt{T/4})] = e^{-cT} \quad (4.16)$$

Hence,

$$\ln\{2[1 - N(\sigma\sqrt{T/4})]\} = -cT \quad (4.17)$$

Or,

$$c = -\ln[2 - 2N(\sigma\sqrt{T/4})]/T \quad (4.18)$$

Because $2[1 - N(\sigma\sqrt{T/4})] = d < 1$, then, $\ln[2 - 2N(\sigma\sqrt{T/4})] < 0$, hence $c = -\ln[2 - 2N(\sigma\sqrt{T/4})]/T > 0$, i.e. c is a positive number. Obviously, Eq. 4.18 is a risk premium model incorporating total risk rather than only systematic risk.

Let k to represent risk adjusted discount rate, and r to represent risk free rate; note that the risk adjusted discount rate is the sum of the time premium and the risk premium, then,

$$k = r + c = r - \ln[2 - 2N(\sigma\sqrt{T/4})]/T \quad (4.19)$$

Of course, as a discount rate, k in Eq. 4.19 incorporates the total risk. To keep in line with the ZZ certainty equivalent related models, we refer to Eqs. 4.18 and 4.19 as ZZ risk premium model and ZZ capital asset pricing model or ZZ CAPM respectively.

4.3.2 Comparison Between Sharpe's CAPM and ZZ CAPM

We now have two models concerning the relationship between risk and return. One is Sharpe's CAPM, which incorporates only the systematic risk; the other is the ZZ CAPM, which incorporates total risk (the systematic risk and the non-systematic risk).

This implies that when we need to determine a discount rate for valuation or financial analyses, we have the flexibility to make a choice between Sharpe's

CAPM and ZZ CAPM. Then, a question is: which is better for determining a discount rate? It is thus necessary to make a systematic comparison between the two models.

Firstly, as we discussed in Chap. 1, finance is a decision-oriented science rather than a descriptive science. As a decision benchmark, what we need in discounting is a required (rate of) return. The required return is neither an ex-post actual one nor a predicted one. Both the ex-post actual return and the predicted return are possible to mismatch with the asset risk; but the required return should theoretically match with the asset risk.

Since Sharpe's CAPM and ZZ CAPM can derive a required return respectively, both are right in this sense. Conceptually, the required return derived by Sharpe's CAPM matches with only part of the asset risk, i.e. the systematic risk; whereas the required return derived by ZZ CAPM matches with the asset's total risk. Normally, for various financial decision-making, what we need to consider is total risk rather than only part risk (regardless it is systematic risk or not). Matching with part risk is equivalent to mismatching with total risk. The Sharpe's CAPM in such sense is not right for determining discount rate.

Secondly, the discount rate derived by the Sharpe's CAPM can be lower than the risk free rate, because the beta of an asset is negative when the asset return is negatively related with other assets. This makes no sense in most circumstances. On the other hand, the discount rate derived by the ZZ CAPM is always higher than the risk free rate, because the risk premium derived by the ZZ risk premium model is always positive. This implies that the ZZ CAPM is sounder in theory and more reliable in practice.

Thirdly, the Sharpe's CAPM takes the diversification effect into consideration; the more securities brought into the portfolio, the more diversification effect, and the lower of the discount rate. While this may make some sense in reality, especially for investment decision in security market; there is another "diversification effect" captured by the ZZ CAPM but neglected by Sharpe's CAPM. The ZZ CAPM incorporates the effect of diversification among periods; the longer the investment lasting, the lower the discount rate should be. This reveals explicitly an almost forgotten principle: the longer of the investment lasting, the lower of its (annual) risk.[4] Hence the successful experience from long-term investment (such as Warren E. Buffett) can be explained by the ZZ CAPM.

Fourthly, it seems that the Sharpe's CAPM and the ZZ CAPM are representing the two extremes. One is full-diversification; the other is zero-diversification in terms of the variety of securities. In fact, the ZZ CAPM can also consider easily the diversification effect across securities. Replacing σ of an asset by σ of the relevant portfolio under consideration, we can easily derive a discount rate matches with the portfolio risk based on the same ZZ CAPM, hence consider the diversification effect properly.

---

[4] Some scholars find that the annual risk premium and the risk-adjusted discount rate should decrease along with the time extending into further future, such as R. Schmalensee [8], M. Weitzman [9], C. Gollier [10], etc.

4.3 Risk Premium and a New CAPM

The model to derive a portfolio variance is as following:

$$\sigma_P^2 = \sum_{i=1}^{n}\sum_{j=1}^{n} w_i w_j \sigma_{i,j} \qquad (4.20)$$

where, w_i, w_j are the weights of the ith and jth assets respectively in the portfolio; $\sigma_{i,j}$ is the co-variance of the returns of the ith and jth assets. Understandingly, when $i = j = x$, $\sigma_{i,j}$ is the variance of the xth assets.

Fifthly, there may be some difficulties in estimating the σ of an asset or the $\sigma_{i,j}$ of two assets, but this should not be a big hurdle in application of the ZZ CAPM. One reason is that the σ of an asset or the $\sigma_{i,j}$ of two assets is already the most basic risk measures in finance. Most risk measures, such as beta, value at risk, etc., are based on the basic variance of assets. The second reason is that the Sharpe's CAPM has been widely used for decades and it (and the beta) relies on the σ of an asset and the $\sigma_{i,j}$ of any two assets heavily. In other words, the application of the Sharpe's CAPM proves the feasibility of the application of the ZZ CAPM in portfolio investment. There are actually many investment and research institutions in the world publish regularly the σ and $\sigma_{i,j}$ of various assets. Anyway, to focus on our core theme, i.e. fundamental financial problems and their solutions, I would not like to further the issue about the estimation of variance and co-variance.

4.3.3 Exemplifications

Again for the example in last section, when the volatility level is 15 % and 25 % respectively, the corresponding c and k are calculated based on the ZZ risk premium model and the ZZ CAPM as shown in Tables 4.6 and 4.7 respectively.

Table 4.6 The estimation of risk adjusted discount rate k (volatility is 15 %)

Years	1	2	3	4	5	6	7	8	9	10
c	0.062	0.044	0.036	0.032	0.029	0.026	0.024	0.023	0.022	0.021
d	0.940	0.916	0.897	0.881	0.867	0.854	0.843	0.832	0.822	0.813
k	0.112	0.094	0.086	0.082	0.079	0.076	0.074	0.073	0.072	0.071
e^{-kT}	0.894	0.828	0.772	0.721	0.675	0.633	0.594	0.558	0.524	0.493

Note e^{-kT} is the discount factor incorporating both systematic and non-systematic risk. The discounting can be divided into risk discounting and time discounting, i.e., $e^{-kT} = e^{-(r+c)T} = e^{-rT}e^{-cT}$; e^{-cT} and e^{-rT} are "risk discount factor" and "time discount factor" respectively

Table 4.7 The estimation of risk adjusted discount rate k (volatility is 25 %)

Years	1	2	3	4	5	6	7	8	9	10
c	0.105	0.076	0.063	0.055	0.050	0.046	0.043	0.040	0.038	0.037
d	0.901	0.860	0.829	0.803	0.780	0.759	0.741	0.724	0.708	0.693
k	0.155	0.126	0.113	0.105	0.100	0.096	0.093	0.090	0.088	0.087
e^{-kT}	0.857	0.778	0.713	0.657	0.607	0.563	0.522	0.485	0.451	0.420

Table 4.8 The consistency of the certainty equivalent and the ZZ CAPM

Years	0	1	2	3	4	5	6	7	8	9	10
Cash flow	−200	10	30	50	70	90	90	70	50	30	10
k		0.155	0.126	0.113	0.105	0.100	0.096	0.093	0.090	0.088	0.087
e^{-kT}	1	0.857	0.778	0.713	0.657	0.607	0.563	0.522	0.485	0.451	0.420
Present value I	−200	8.57	23.34	35.66	46.00	54.66	50.64	36.55	24.25	13.54	4.20
CE	−200	9.01	25.79	41.43	56.18	70.19	68.35	51.86	36.18	21.23	6.93
e^{-rT}	1	0.951	0.905	0.861	0.819	0.779	0.741	0.705	0.670	0.638	0.607
Present value II	−200	8.57	23.34	35.66	46.00	54.66	50.64	36.55	24.25	13.54	4.20

In Tables 4.6 and 4.7, the c, or the annual risk premium rate as well as the risk-adjusted discount rate, decreases as the due time goes on. As explained above, this is because the investment is better time-diversified as the number of period increases; more and more risks are canceled out among periods. Nevertheless, the certainty coefficient still keeps decreasing from year to year; similarly, the total discount factor, e^{-kT}, calculated based on the total discount rate k, also remains decreasing from year to year. This implies that the further in future of a variable, the larger part of its value is discounted out or the smaller part of its value remains as present value. This obviously makes sense.

Please note that the ZZ models of certainty equivalent and its coefficient, the ZZ models of risk equivalent and its coefficient, the ZZ risk premium model and the ZZ CAPM are mutually consistent in logic. In other words, we'll get the same result either via discounting the certainty equivalent at the risk free rate or via discounting the predicted cash flow at the risk adjusted discount rate. For example, for the volatility level of 25 %, the discounting results of the cash flows from project G via the two methods are shown in Table 4.8.

Please note in Table 4.8, present value I and present value II are identical. Present value I (the fifth row) results from discounting the predicted cash flow at the risk adjusted discount rate, i.e. predicted cash flow multiplied by e^{-kT}, while present value II (the bottom row) results from discounting the certainty equivalent at the risk free rate, i.e. certainty equivalent multiplied by e^{-rT}. Obviously, the certainty equivalent model or certainty coefficient model and the risk premium model or CAPM are mutually consistent.

4.4 Summary

We now solve the fundamental problem of incorporating total risk into required return or discount rate as well as into asset valuation or financial decisions with a series of models: the ZZ models of certainty equivalent and its coefficient, the ZZ risk equivalent and its coefficient, the ZZ risk premium model and the ZZ CAPM.

4.4 Summary

Neither the forms nor the variables of these models are chosen subjectively, just like the model series of stock valuation and theoretical ratios in last chapter. In other words, both the forms and the variables of these models are derived via strict logic processes. Also similar to the innovative models in last chapter, the models in this chapter are simple in form and feasible in practice, hence will benefit the related financial calculations, such as the estimation of the certainty equivalent as well as the risk-adjusted discount rate, etc. As the important and fundamental innovations, these models will support more effectively the related financial decisions, such as investment decision, stock valuation and asset pricing as well as risk management.

References

1. Sharpe WF (1964) Capital asset prices: a theory of market equilibrium under conditions of risk. J Financ 19(3):425–442
2. Gordon AS (1986) A certainty–equivalent approach to capital budgeting. Financ Manage 15(4):23–32
3. Becker JL, Sarin RK (1987) Lottery dependent utility. Manage Sci 33:1367–1382
4. Gollier C, Pratt JW (1996) Risk vulnerability and the tempering effect of background risk. Econometrica 64(6):1109–1123
5. Rabin M (2000) Risk aversion and expected–utility theory: a calibration theorem. Econometrica 68(6):1281–1292
6. Hennessy DA, Lapan HE (2006) On the nature of certainty equivalent functionals. J Math Econ 43(1):1–10
7. Turner AL, Weigel EJ (1992) Daily stock market volatility: 1928–1989. Manage Sci 38(11):1586–1609
8. Schmalensee R (1981) Risk and return on long–lived tangible assets. J Financ Econ 185–205
9. Weitzman M (1998) Why the far distant future should be discounted at its lowest possible rate. J Environ Econ Manage 36:201–208
10. Gollier C (2002) Time horizon and the discount rate. J Econ Theor 107(3):463–73

Chapter 5
Tax Shield, Bankruptcy Cost and Optimal Capital Structure

Capital is a must for every firm. The capitals backing of businesses include debt and equity. Firms raise their capitals in capital market. When firms make their financing decision, they have to consider the problem of capital structure, i.e. the mix of equity and debt, which is often represented by the debt ratio, or referred to as leverage ratio.

The optimal debt ratio is the debt ratio that can maximize a firm's value. Modigliani and Miller reveal very important insights about capital structure, but they fail to solve the problem of optimal capital structure. This chapter derives an optimal capital structure model based on the trade off between the main cost and benefit of debt, i.e. the tax shield and bankruptcy cost, thus solve the problem of optimal capital structure.

5.1 Firm's Goal and its Capital Structure

The fundamental goal of a firm is to maximize its value through various decisions, which mainly include investment decision, financing decision and operating decision. As for financing decision, a practical and meaningful question is: can we increase a firm's value by adjusting its capital structure? How? This is involving the issue of optimal capital structure.

The problem of optimal capital structure has been intensively studied since MM model Modigliani and Miller [1, 2], but has not been effectively solved. That is, scholars have not developed a theoretically sound model of optimal capital structure. Firms in reality thus have to make their capital structure decisions intuitively.

A common way to make a decision is to choose the best (optimal) one among all available alternatives via trading-off between the potential benefits and costs. As for capital structure decision, similarly, an optimal debt ratio can be determined by trading-off between the potential benefits and costs related to the debt financing.[1] From the MM model I to the trade-off theory, the conventional research of capital structure goes along this way.

Thus, the problem of capital structure decision is equivalent to: what is the optimal debt ratio? To solve such a problem, we should know: what are the potential benefits and costs of debt financing and how do they change along with the increasing or decreasing of the debt ratio? Understandingly, the optimal capital structure is the debt ratio where the net benefit of the debt financing is maximized, or the firm value is maximized.

Note that solving any problem need to assume other things being equal. To solve the problem of optimal capital structure, we should assume that other aspects of the firm, such as the business and investment as well as the size of total asset, are unchanged. While there are numerous comprehensive researches in this area, the problem of primary importance still is: other things being equal, what is the optimal debt ratio of the firm?

5.2 The Potential Benefits and Costs of Debt Financing

There is a wide variety of potential benefits and costs related to the debt financing. However, as a common sense, for the convenience and efficiency in actual financial decision, we should focus on the benefits and costs with direct and great importance.

5.2.1 General Analyses

When a firm uses debt capital, it is obliged to repay the due interests and principle at the maturity of the debt, hence has the risk of default or bankruptcy. Because of this, from investors' point of view, debt (such as corporate bond) is safer than equity. This leads to the investors' required rate of return on debt is lower than that on equity. The investors' required rate of return determines the cost of capital borne by the borrowing firm. Therefore, from the firms' point of view, debt financing has a benefit of lower cost and a cost of bankruptcy risk. The cost arising from bankruptcy risk is often referred to as bankruptcy cost; and the usage of debt capital is often referred to as usage of financial leverage.

There is another important difference between debt and equity. As a worldwide rule, the cost of debt, including the interests and price discount, is paid as a cost. Such a cost is paid before corporate (income) tax, hence deducted from the

---

[1] You can also choose an optimal equity size or ratio by trading-off the potential benefits and costs related to the equity financing. This is equivalent to the consideration from the debt side which is the academic convention.

firm's income. Oppositely, the cost of equity, similarly including the dividends and price discount, is paid after corporate tax hence deducted from the firm's earnings. In other words, the cost of debt is treated as a real cost, but the cost of equity is treated as a part of earnings. Thus firms can get corporate tax savings from debt capital. This is another benefit of debt in addition to the lower capital cost, which is referred to as tax shield in the arena of capital structure.

In summary, debt financing has two important benefits including the lower cost and the tax shield and one important cost referred to as the bankruptcy cost.

5.2.2 MM Model I

In 1958, Modigliani and Miller publish their breakthrough papers concerning firms' capital structure decision. They reveal that, in an assumed environment without corporate tax and bankruptcy risk, a firm's value is irrelevant to its debt ratio. Meanwhile, they reveal that the firm's weighted average cost of capital (WACC) is also irrelevant to its debt ratio.[2] These relationships are shown in Eq. 5.1:

$$V_L = EBIT/WACC = EBIT/K_{SU} = V_U \qquad (5.1)$$

Where V_L is the levered firm value; EBIT is the annual earnings before interest and tax; WACC is the weighted average cost of capital in the levered firm; K_{SU} is the cost of equity in unlevered firm; V_U is the unlevered firm value. Obviously, firm L and firm U are only different in capital mix, i.e., one is levered, the other is unlevered.

The reasoning behind the irrelevance of capital structure or Eq. 5.1 is: as the debt ratio increases, the earnings left over (after paying interests or cost to debt investors) to equity investors is down-sizing and more volatile; hence the required rate of return on equity or the cost of equity capital is increasing. The increase in equity cost will just cancel out the cost reduction effect from the debt financing. Therefore, it is useless if a firm tries to lower its WACC or to raise its value by adjusting the debt ratio, because the increase in low-cost debt is always followed by the increase in the equity cost.

---

[2] We reveal in Chap. 4 (4.1 Alternatives to determine a discount rate) that the discount rate is different from the cost of capital (including the weighted average cost of capital, WACC), because the capital cost is the result of financing (decision), and may have nothing to do with the asset risk. The discount rate is the investors' benchmark to value an asset (such as a project or firm etc.), and has much to do with the asset risk. However, financial scholars are used to refer to the discount rate as capital cost (including the WACC and the equity cost) in the discussion of capital structure since Modigliani and Miller. We continue to use such an appellation in this chapter to avoid unnecessary chaos or difficulties for readers. Nevertheless, readers should aware that the WACC and the equity cost in this chapter is the appropriate WACC and the appropriate equity cost, which incorporate the relevant risk and can be used as the discount rate to derive the value of the firm and its equity respectively. In other words, the cost of capital in this chapter is exactly the fair cost of capital or discount rate rather than the actual cost of capital.

Modigliani and Miller's finding in 1958 is afterwards referred to as MM model I or the irrelevance of capital structure. Please note that MM model I has not eliminated the possibility of increasing firm value via optimizing its capital structure, because their conclusion is derived in an assumed environment without corporate tax and bankruptcy risk, which is significantly different from the reality. Nevertheless, MM model I is very important because it implies that the benefit of low-cost from debt is not an achievable benefit, thus the debt financing actually has only one important benefit, i.e. the tax shield. In other words, the cheapness of debt is no longer a benefit worthy to consider in capital structure decisions.

Thanks to Modigliani and Miller, because of their contribution, to solve the problem of optimal capital structure, we need not to care about the cheapness of debt. All we should focus on are the tax shield and the bankruptcy cost, or on how to maximize the difference between the tax shield and the bankruptcy cost.

5.3 Efforts to Value Tax Shield and Bankruptcy Cost

MM model I casts light on the problem of optimal capital structure. During the years after it, scholars focus on the valuation of tax shield and the bankruptcy cost.

5.3.1 MM Model II

In 1963, Modigliani and Miller relax the condition of no corporate tax in MM model I and publish a new model incorporating the tax shield. They denote the corporate tax rate by T, the size of debt by D, and the cost of debt by i, then the annual tax savings is DTi. Assume the annual tax savings are perpetual cash flows and the appropriate discount rate is i, its value then is $DTi/i = DT$. Eq. 5.1 is then rewritten as:

$$V_L = V_U + DT \tag{5.2}$$

Equation 5.2 is referred to as MM model II. Modigliani and Miller fail to find an effective way to value the bankruptcy cost hence still cannot incorporate the bankruptcy cost into their new model. Unsurprisingly, with only the benefit (tax shield) taken into account, the derived optimal debt ratio is 100 % based on the new model. This is again an unpractical conclusion.

Neither MM model I nor MM model II is the final solution to the problem of optimal capital structure. Anyway, MM Model I and II open a new era of research on optimal capital structure. Modigliani and Miller win the Nobel Prize in 1985 and 1990 respectively for their contributions to finance and economics. After that, more and more scholars try to quantify the bankruptcy cost but get no satisfied solution. Therefore, the optimal capital structure remains unsolved in theory, and firms have to make their capital structure decisions intuitively.

5.3.2 The Trade-Off Model

Since MM model II, some scholars emphasize that the optimal leverage ratio should be derived by trading-off between the benefits and costs of debt, such as Kraus and Litzenberger [3], DeAngelo and Masulis [4], Robichek and Myers (1966), Scott (1976) etc. They are referred to as the school of trade-off theory in finance. Unfortunately, they fail to model the bankruptcy cost either, and even fail to value the tax shield correctly.

Figure 5.1 is a typical demonstration of scholars' expectation based on the conventional trade-off theory. In the absent of bankruptcy cost, the firm value will increase proportionally with the debt ratio, just as what depicted in the MM model II. In reality, as the debt ratio increases, the actual firm value increases because of the increase of the tax shield; and then increases slowly because of the faster increase of the bankruptcy cost; and then decreases because the bankruptcy cost increases over the tax shield. The firm value goes firstly upwards and then downwards; the top point is the optimum of the capital structure.

In prevailing finance books, the trade-off model is usually written as:

$$V_L = V_U + DT - \text{bankruptcy cost} \tag{5.3}$$

The "DT" in Eq. 5.3 is copied from the MM model II. As mentioned earlier, MM model II derives the tax shield as "DT" under the assumption of no bankruptcy risk; hence the firm and its tax savings of "DTi" can last forever. However, the trade-off model attempts to remedy the MM model II, i.e. to consider additionally the bankruptcy cost. Obviously, with the existence of potential bankruptcy, the annual tax savings can no longer last forever, and the value of the tax shield should be much lower than "DT".

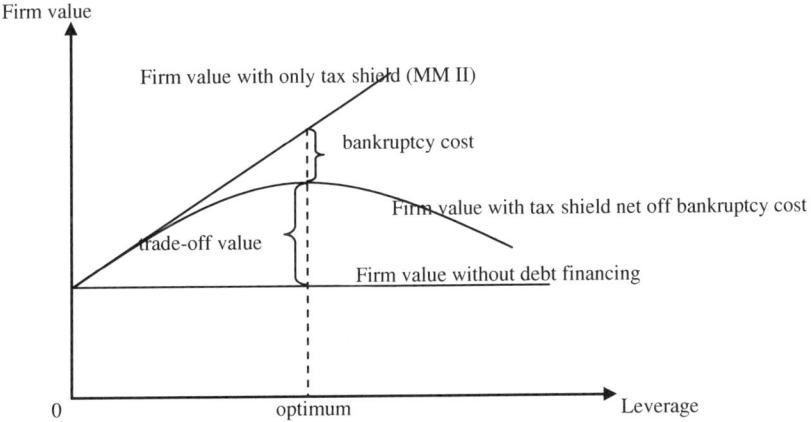

Fig. 5.1 Traditional expectation of the value-addition from capital structure

Therefore, the trade-off model contradicts itself. On one hand, it tries to incorporate the bankruptcy cost; on the other hand, it assumes the tax savings of the firm can last forever. Such a conceptual error (self-contradictory) has not been recognized; most prevailing financial textbooks are copying and propagating such a trade-off model.

There are more discussions on valuing the tax shield after MM model II and traditional trade-off theory, such as Kane, Marcus and McDonald [5], Miles and Ezzell [6], Graham [7], Arzac and Glosten (2005), Cooper and Nyborg [8], etc. Graham [7] estimates the capitalized tax benefits of debt to be as high as 5 % of firm value. Recently, Korteweg [9] derives that the median firm captures net benefits of up to 5.5 % of firm value at its optimal leverage ratio. Van Binsbergen, Graham and Yang [10] estimate that the gross and net benefits of debt are 10.4 and 3.5 % of asset value respectively.

Unfortunately, most (if not all) of the studies focus on empirical evidence from past data and reveal little decision- or future- oriented insight. Actually, a tax shield number (rather than a model) cannot be useful for finding an optimal debt ratio.

5.3.3 Other Efforts

Besides the tax shield, there are even more misunderstandings on the bankruptcy cost in prior research. Within the context of optimal capital structure, bankruptcy cost by prevailing definition includes direct and indirect costs. The direct costs include items like legal, accounting, and other professional fees, firm reorganization costs, etc. The indirect costs include those like lost sales resulted from falling demand, declining margins resulted from various increased input costs, loss of key personnel and the additional input of management time and effort.[3]

The indirect costs are difficult to value and consequently, most prior studies of bankruptcy cost focus on the direct costs. For instance, Warner (1977) investigates 11 bankrupt railroad companies, and estimates that direct bankruptcy costs are 5.3 % of firm value. Based on a sample of 37 companies, Iiss (1990) estimates that direct bankruptcy costs are 3.1 % of firm value. Based on 212 firms filing for bankruptcy in New York and Arizona, Bris, llch and Zhu (2006) estimate this ratio is about 9.5 %.

There are indeed some scholars making efforts to estimate the indirect bankruptcy cost, such as Haugen and Senbet (1988), Andrade and Kaplan [11]. Based on 31 highly levered firms, Andrade and Kaplan [11] estimate that the cost of financial distress[4] is about 10 % to 20 % of firm value. Recently, Bhamra et al. (2008) and Chen [12] try to estimate the cost of default of the investment grade firms and speculative grade firms respectively. Van Binsbergen, Graham and Yang 10 estimate gross cost of debt equal to 6.9 % of asset value.

---

[3] There are some relevant prevailing terminologies, such as debt overhang (Myers 1977), asset substitution (Jensen and Meckling 1976), and asset fire-sales (Shleifer and Vishny 1992), etc.

[4] Basically, financial distress cost is only a new name of indirect bankruptcy cost.

5.3 Efforts to Value Tax Shield and Bankruptcy Cost

Again, a bankruptcy cost number (rather than a model) cannot be helpful for finding an optimal debt ratio. In addition, the direct bankruptcy costs are the transaction costs of the actual bankruptcy, whereas the indirect costs are the real bankruptcy costs. The indirect costs occur far earlier and more frequently and are likely larger than the direct costs. In most circumstances, the firm remains healthy until and beyond the debt maturity and the direct costs will not eventually occur, but the indirect costs will surely occur, more or less. If we cannot measure the indirect costs, we actually cannot measure the real bankruptcy costs.

Even worse, the conventional division of bankruptcy costs——direct and indirect ones are the ex post concepts. Related to such concepts, most (if not all) researchers estimate the indirect bankruptcy costs based on sample data. However, decision is always forward looking; capital structure decision is not an exception. Therefore, capital structure as well as other financial models should be ex-ante models rather than a backward looking or ex-post descriptive models. For healthy firms to make their capital structure decisions, what they need is a model relating the bankruptcy cost to the debt size or ratio, rather than a simple estimated number of bankruptcy cost based on some past data. It seems impossible to quantify the bankruptcy cost correctly based on the prevailing concepts.

As an ex-ante concept, the bankruptcy cost should be a present value of the expected possible future costs rather than actual costs in statistics. Since debt financing increases the bankruptcy risk and consequently reduce the firm value, we define bankruptcy cost as the firm value reduction now resulted from the future potential bankruptcy risk.[5] Such a definition reflects the important features of this cost, i.e. the contingency and the uncertainty.

5.4 Decision-Oriented Valution of Tax Shield and Bankruptcy Cost

After revising the conceptual errors on tax shield and bankruptcy cost, we focus on the valuation of them in this section in case of potential bankruptcy.

5.4.1 The Time Horizon

MM models (I and II) follow an assumption of no bankruptcy risk, so they value the relevant benefits and costs over an infinite period. In reality, however, a firm will surely go bankrupt over an infinite or long enough period. As a common case, when a firm goes bankrupt, its value falls below its debt book value and its equity value falls to zero.

---

[5] This may be close to the prevailing concept of distress cost, which may includes also agency cost, etc., but I will not distinguish those costs in detail, and just regard them as all aroused from the debt financing.

Therefore, from the firm owner's (equity-holder's) point, considering over an infinite or long enough time horizon, avoiding bankruptcy definitely outweighs obtaining the tax shield. In such a sense, the optimal capital structure is definitely 0 % debt or 100 % equity, rather than 100 % debt as predicted by MM model II. Of course, neither 100 % equity nor 100 % debt is the "right" solution for capital structure decision. The two extreme "optimal" debt ratios just reflect that the infinite period is a wrong choice of time horizon for the capital structure decision and we cannot get an effective solution this way.

The time horizon has received little attention in previous research on capital structure; but the fundamental difference between practical decision and academic assumption in the time horizon may be one of the key reasons that the optimal capital structure remains unsolved. A convincing evidence is that no managers base their (capital structure) decisions on infinite future even they do not care their tenures. So we should choose a more practical time horizon as the first step for solving the problem of optimal capital structure.

Along with the growth of a firm, it will finance round by round; capital structure decision is among the considerations of every round of financing. When a firm considers its capital structure, what it should care about is the benefits and costs of the debt determined by the current round financing, rather than those benefits and costs determined by last round financing or next round financing or financing in the distant future.

Thus, it is natural and correct to trade-off between tax shield and bankruptcy cost on the basis of the current financing round. The time before next round financing is usually determined by a firm's growth opportunity and/or its debt maturity. Most people caring a firm, whether they are insiders or outsiders, are aware easily of the firm's debt maturity; but they seldom know the time of the next financing round of the firm arising from a growth opportunity. In addition, growth opportunity is not directly related to bankruptcy, while repaying of debt principal is usually a direct cause of bankruptcy.[6] Therefore, to make things relatively simple and certain, the best choice of time horizon for the purpose of capital structure decision should be the debt maturity determined by the current round financing.

We thus redefine the problem of optimal capital structure as: the debt ratio maximizing the difference between the tax shield and the bankruptcy cost during the debt life.

5.4.2 Value the Tax Shield

Now we consider how to value the tax shield during the debt life determined by the current round financing. We use S and X to denote the current market value of

---

[6] Some scholars study the capital structure decision with possible bankruptcy before the debt maturity, such as Ju et al. [13]. For the general validity and decisional efficiency of the solution, I will focus on the most simple and common situation, where the bankruptcy can only occur at the debt maturity.

5.4 Decision-Oriented Valution of Tax Shield and Bankruptcy Cost

a firm and its debt respectively. The firm's debt or leverage ratio then is X/S. For a healthy firm, the debt market value is close to its book value. So we assume the initial market value of the debt is also its book value and is the base for calculating the interest payment.

A firm usually has various debts. Debts with maturity less than one year are current debts or short term debts among which the most common part is payables; debts with maturity longer than one year are long term debts. X in this chapter denotes all debts a firm owes, including short term debt and long term debt. Some research only considers long term debt with reasoning that most short term debts (such as payables) bear no interest cost hence will not contribute tax shield. However, the short term debts still "contribute" bankruptcy risk or bankruptcy cost just as the long term debt does. We thus have to take all short term and long term debts into account in valuing bankruptcy cost. For this reason, we should not neglect the short term debts in valuing tax shield, because we should definitely consider the identical debt when we trade-off between its tax shield and its bankruptcy cost.

Besides the debt size, the debt tax shield depends also on the interest rate, the time to maturity and the corporate tax rate. To make things simple, use b and T to represent the average interest rate and the average maturity of all short term and long term debts, and f to represent the corporate (income) tax rate. Define the perpetual tax shield as the tax shield of the debts over an infinite time horizon in absent of bankruptcy, just as the DT in MM model II. Thanks to MM model II, the perpetual tax shield of the debts starting from now is:

$$\frac{Xbf}{b} = Xf \quad (5.4)$$

Where Xf is equivalent to DT in MM model II.

Following a convention in financial research, let r to denote the annual risk free rate and assume all asset values are compounding continuously at r. Then the present value of the perpetual tax shield starting from the debt (future) maturity is:

$$\frac{Xbf}{b}e^{-rT} = Xfe^{-rT} \quad (5.5)$$

Therefore, value of the tax shield (TS) during the debt life is (5.4)–(5.5):

$$TS = Xf - Xfe^{-rT} = Xf\left(1 - e^{-rT}\right) \quad (5.6)$$

Where, X is the book value and current market value of the firm's debt; f is the corporate tax rate; r is the risk free rate; T is the maturity of the firm's debt. Since Eq. 5.6 is different from other theoretical and empirical tax shield model, for the convenience to be referred to, I would like to name it as ZZ tax shield model.

Let's test the ZZ tax shield model via applying it to a numerical example. Assume a typical base case, where the value of the firm and its debt is 100 and 50 respectively, the corporate tax rate $f = 30\%$, the risk free rate $r = 3.0\%$, the average debt maturity $T = 4$. Based on Eq. 5.6, the ZZ tax shield (present value) over the debt life is,

TS = 50 × 30 % × (1−e$^{-3\% \times 4}$) = 1.6962

For the same case, the MM tax shield over infinite tome horizon is,

TS$_{MM}$ = 50 × 30 % = 15

For the same case, the MM tax shield is 15 % of the firm value, whereas the ZZ tax shield is only 1.6962 % of the firm value. This demonstrates the significant difference between the MM tax shield and the ZZ tax shield. An interesting question is: which one is correct? It should not be difficult for you to find the right answer to this question.

As other ZZ models in previous chapters, the ZZ tax shield model is derived based on correct concepts and strict logic rather than chosen subjectively in terms of its form and the variables incorporated. In addition, the ZZ tax shield model also makes sense because the relationships among the relevant variables revealed in the model are completely in line with common intuitions. For instance, the tax shield should be positively related with the debt size (X) and its maturity (T), corporate tax rate (f) and the risk free rate (r).[7] These relationships are all reflected in the ZZ tax shield model or Eq. 5.6.

5.4.3 Value the Bankruptcy Cost

The value of the debt, compounding continuously at r, is expected to be FV(X) = Xe^{rT} on its maturity. As shown in Fig. 5.2, on the maturity date, if the firm value is larger than Xe^{rT}, the firm keeps healthy and the debt value is Xe^{rT} (represented by the right part of the dash line); if the firm value is smaller than Xe^{rT}, the firm will go bankrupt. In such a case, the firm cannot afford to repay all debts with its assets; the debt value equals to the firm value (less than Xe^{rT} and represented by the left part of the dash line); and the equity value falls to zero.

Thus the bankruptcy risk can be represented by the left part of the dash line in Fig. 5.2 when the firm and its debt value fall below Xe^{rT} at the debt maturity. A put option can hedge such a risk exactly. As shown in Fig. 5.2, a put option with exercise price of Xe^{rT} and maturity as the debt maturity (represented by the black line) cancels out the bankruptcy risk exactly and guarantees the debt value not lower than Xe^{rT}, or change the risky debt into a risk free debt (represented by the horizontal line in Fig. 5.2).

Since the put option is just enough to save the debt from bankruptcy risk, the value or cost of the put option is just the bankruptcy cost.[8] According to the most common cases, we assume bankruptcy can only occur at the debt maturity, thus the option to hedge the bankruptcy risk is a standard European put option with maturity T. Thanks to Black and Scholes (1973), Merton (1973), as shown in Chap. 3, the value of such a put option is:

---

[7] Note that the risk free rate is positively related with the interest rate of the debt.

[8] See also Graya et al. [14].

5.4 Decision-Oriented Valuation of Tax Shield and Bankruptcy Cost

Fig. 5.2 Bankruptcy cost = put option

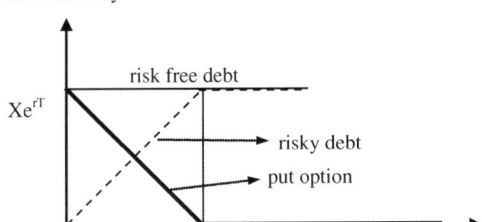

$$\text{put} = Xe^{-rT}N(-d2) - SN(-d1) \tag{5.7}$$

Where, N(−d2) and N(−d1) are the cumulative probabilities under standard normal distribution when the Z values equal to −d2 and −d1 respectively, and:

$$d1 = \frac{\ln(S/X) + (r + \sigma^2/2)T}{\sigma\sqrt{T}} \tag{5.8}$$

$$d2 = \frac{\ln(S/X) + (r - \sigma^2/2)T}{\sigma\sqrt{T}} = d1 - \sigma\sqrt{T} \tag{5.9}$$

Where σ is the standard deviation of annual return (the relative dividend and value change) of the stock (underlying asset). Since the underlying asset S now is the firm value, σ here is the standard deviation of the relative value change of the firm.

Please note that X in the standard Black–Scholes-Merton option pricing model (Eqs. 5.7–5.9) is the exercise price of the option, i.e. a future value at the maturity of the option, whereas X in this chapter is defined as the present value of the debt, hence X in this chapter is equivalent to Xe^{-rT} in the standard option pricing model. Please also note that $\ln(S/X) + rT = \ln[S/(Xe^{-rT})]$ and $(\sigma^2/2)T/(\sigma\sqrt{T}) = \sigma\sqrt{T}/2$. Thus, replacing the Xe^{-rT} in Eq. 5.7, 5.8 and 5.9 by X, the model of the bankruptcy cost (BC) is:

$$BC = XN(-d2) - SN(-d1) \tag{5.10}$$

Where, S and X are the current market value of the firm and its debt respectively, and,

$$d1 = \frac{\ln(S/X)}{\sigma\sqrt{T}} + \frac{\sigma\sqrt{T}}{2} \tag{5.11}$$

$$d2 = \frac{\ln(S/X)}{\sigma\sqrt{T}} - \frac{\sigma\sqrt{T}}{2} = d1 - \sigma\sqrt{T} \tag{5.12}$$

Where, σ is the standard deviation of the relative change in the firm value; T is the average maturity of all debts owned by the firm.

Since Eq. 5.10 (and the related Eqs. 5.11 and 5.12) is different from other theoretical and empirical bankruptcy cost model, for the convenience to be referred to, I would like to name it as ZZ bankruptcy cost model.

Let's test the ZZ bankruptcy cost model via applying it to the previous typical base case, where the value of the firm and its debt is 100 and 50 respectively, the corporate tax rate f = 30 %, the risk free rate r = 3.0 %, the average debt maturity T = 4, the volatility of the return on total assets of the firm σ = 26 %.[9] Based on Eq. 5.10–5.12, the ZZ bankruptcy cost (present value) over the debt life is calculated as following,

$$d1 = \frac{\ln(100/50)}{26\%\sqrt{4}} + \frac{26\%\sqrt{4}}{2} = 1.5930$$

$$d2 = \frac{\ln(100/50)}{26\%\sqrt{4}} - \frac{26\%\sqrt{4}}{2} = 1.0730$$

$$N(-d1) = 0.0556$$

$$N(-d2) = 0.1416$$

$$BC = 1.5238$$

Now the ZZ bankruptcy cost is 1.5238, or the bankruptcy cost is about 1.5238 % of the firm value. As calculated earlier, the corresponding tax shield is 1.6962 % of the firm value. This implies the net benefit of the debt financing is only 0.17 % of the firm value. As the firm now has 50 % debt in its total capital, an interesting question is: does the very small net benefit (0.17 % of the firm value) imply the firm over levered or under levered? This question may be not easy to answer as it seems to be now; but will be very easy to answer after you read the next section (Sect. 5.5).

As other previous ZZ models, the ZZ bankruptcy cost model is derived based on correct concepts and strict logic rather than chosen subjectively in terms of its form and the variables incorporated. In addition, the ZZ bankruptcy cost model also makes sense because the relationships among the relevant variables revealed in the model are completely in line with intuitions. For instance, the bankruptcy probability hence bankruptcy cost should be positively related with the debt size (X) and its maturity (T) as well as the firm value volatility (σ), and negatively related with the firm value (S).[10] These relationships are all reflected in the ZZ bankruptcy cost model or Eq. 5.10–5.12.

---

[9] Most researches on capital structure choose 20 % as the typical volatility; but some choose a value close to 40 %, such as Ju et al. [13], etc. Here I just choose a value somewhere in between.

[10] These relationships will be more easily to be understood when they related to the payoff or intrinsic value and time value of the relevant put option.

5.5 Decision-Oriented Optimal Capital Structure Model

5.5.1 Derivation of the Model

Combining Eqs. 5.6 and 5.10, or subtracting the bankruptcy cost from the tax shield, we can get the ZZ trade–off value or the net benefit of the debt financing:

$$\begin{aligned} \text{ZZ Trade-off value} &= \text{Net benefit of debt financing} \\ &= \text{Tax shield–Bankruptcy cost} \\ &= Xf\left(1 - e^{-rT}\right) - [XN(-d2) - SN(-d1)] \end{aligned} \quad (5.13)$$

Mathematically, when the derivative of Eq. 5.13 with respect to X equals to zero, the capital structure reaches its optimum. The condition that the derivative equals to zero is shown as Eq. 5.14 with detailed derivation shown in Appendix at the end of this chapter.

$$N(-d2) = f\left(1 - e^{-rT}\right) \quad (5.14)$$

Denote the debt or leverage ratio (capital structure) as $L = X/S$, then $\ln(S/X) = \ln(1/L) = -\ln(L)$. Based on Eq. 5.12,

$$-d2 = -\frac{\ln(S/X)}{\sigma\sqrt{T}} + \frac{\sigma\sqrt{T}}{2} = \frac{\ln(L)}{\sigma\sqrt{T}} + \frac{\sigma\sqrt{T}}{2}$$

Thus, Eq. 5.14 can be rewritten as:

$$N\left[\frac{\ln(L)}{\sigma\sqrt{T}} + \frac{\sigma\sqrt{T}}{2}\right] = f\left(1 - e^{-rT}\right) \quad (5.15)$$

The leverage (or debt) ratio L satisfying Eq. 5.15 is obviously the optimal leverage ratio. It is easy to find the L based on Eq. 5.15 by using of the "goal seek" function in Excel. So we solve the problem of optimal capital structure.

We can also resort the inverse cumulative distribution function or "probit function" to "solve out" the "L" in Eq. 5.15. Conceptually, $\text{probit}(p) = N^{-1}(p)$, $\text{probit}[N(p)] = p$, thus, "probit" the two sides of Eq. 5.15,

$$\frac{\ln(L)}{\sigma\sqrt{T}} + \frac{\sigma\sqrt{T}}{2} = \text{probit}\left[f\left(1 - e^{-rT}\right)\right] \quad (5.16)$$

$$\begin{aligned} \ln(L) &= \{\text{probit}\left[f\left(1 - e^{-rT}\right)\right] - \frac{\sigma\sqrt{T}}{2}\}\sigma\sqrt{T} \\ &= \left[\text{probit}\left(f - fe^{-rT}\right)\right]\sigma\sqrt{T} - \sigma^2 T/2 \end{aligned} \quad (5.17)$$

Then,

$$\begin{aligned}L &= e^{[probit(f-fe^{-rT})]\sigma\sqrt{T}-\sigma^2 T/2}\\ &= \exp\left\{[\text{probit}(f-fe^{-rT})]\sigma\sqrt{T}-\sigma^2 T/2\right\}\end{aligned} \quad (5.18)$$

Eqs. 5.15 or 5.18 provide a clear way to derive optimal leverage or optimal capital structure based on the ZZ tax shield and ZZ bankruptcy cost. I thus name them as ZZ optimal leverage or optimal capital structure condition and model respectively; and refer to the ZZ tax shield model, ZZ bankruptcy cost model, the ZZ optimal leverage condition and the ZZ optimal leverage model as ZZ model series on leverage. Both the condition and the model are the innovative solutions to the problem of optimal capital structure which has been remained unsolved for at least 50 years since MM models. It is convenient to use the "NORMSINV" function in Excel to derive the result of the function probit(). So Eq. 5.18 is a practical or feasible way to find the optimal leverage ratio.

Now, for any given firm, based on the reliable estimates of the conditional variables, including the corporate tax rate f, the debt maturity T, the risk free interest rate r and the volatility of the firm value σ, we can determine its optimal debt or leverage ratio. One thing worthy to mention is that the optimal debt ratio derived through the ZZ leverage model is a ratio based on market values of the debt and equity rather than their book values, which is in line with the tradition in capital structure research.

Consider again the previous base case firm, where the corporate tax rate f = 30 %; the risk free rate r = 3.0 %; the debt maturity T = 4; the return volatility σ = 26 %. The optimal debt ratio of the firm can be derived easily by applying the ZZ optimal leverage model, i.e., L = 33.80 % rounding to two decimals. Hence the firm now is over levered (actual debt ratio is 50 % and actual trade-off value is 0.17). This optimal leverage ratio (33.80 %) is close to many survey data, which implies that the intuitions of all firms' decision-makers on average are roughly unbiased for their leverage choices.

5.5.2 Basic Features of the Model

The ZZ leverage model takes four independent variables into account, i.e. the corporate tax rate (f), the risk free rate (r), the debt maturity (T) as well as the firm value volatility (σ). Again, as all previous ZZ models, the ZZ leverage model is derived based on correct concepts and strict logic rather than chosen subjectively in terms of its form and the variables incorporated. Comparing with other capital structure models so far, the ZZ leverage model has several advantages, which include but do not limit to:

(1) It solves the problem of optimal capital structure clearly and definitely via trading-off between the core cost and benefit of debt capital (tax shield and bankruptcy cost), rather than just describe the results or special data of actual capital structure decisions which is equivocal in properness or not necessarily correct or optimal.

5.5 Decision-Oriented Optimal Capital Structure Model

(2) The derivation goes along a common and simple idea: trading off between the main benefit and cost of debt capital via rigorous logic process. The main benefit and cost of debt financing are the tax shield and bankruptcy cost respectively. So the final optimal model is based on the properly modeling of the tax shield and bankruptcy cost.

(3) Correct concepts are essential for solve financial problems. The concepts of the tax shield and bankruptcy cost in prevailing capital structure research is not correct in terms of time horizon. The ZZ leverage model is derived based on a correct time horizon, i.e. the periods extending to the debt maturity determined by the financing under consideration.

(4) The ZZ leverage model is based on the most essential and simple assumptions, such as the existence of both corporate tax and bankruptcy risk; other details are assumed as simple as possible so long as they are roughly realistic, such as that bankruptcy is assumed only possible at debt maturity. This is necessary for a fundamental solution which should be flexible enough for adjustments in various special applications.

(5) All the variables incorporated in the ZZ leverage model are the direct and important determinants of the optimal capital structure. While numerous factors have some influences on a firm's capital structure decision, some of them are indirectly related to the decision, such as the industry that the firm operating in, the firm's business strategy, market competition, macroeconomic factors, etc.; some of them are unimportant factors, such as the personality as well as the education and other background of the decision makers, etc.

Most of the important indirect factors are actually incorporated into the model via the four direct variables. For instance, the factors related to future market and macro economy conditions are reflected in the current firm value (S) and its volatility (σ).

Some of the prior studies include bankruptcy probability in their models in the sense that the higher the bankruptcy probability the larger the bankruptcy cost. Actually, the bankruptcy probability is implied already in the volatility of the firm's value and the debt maturity. As a common sense, the bankruptcy probability is positively related with the volatility of the firm's value and the debt maturity. This is obviously in line with what indicated by the ZZ bankruptcy cost model, i.e., the bankruptcy cost is also positively related with the volatility of the firm's value and the debt maturity; This is also in line with the ZZ optimal leverage model in which the optimal debt ratio is negative related with the volatility of the firm's value and the debt maturity. It is thus not necessary to further incorporate the bankruptcy probability into the model. In addition, as an independent variable, the bankruptcy probability is too difficult to estimate objectively for a healthy firm. No one can judge the quality of the estimation even afterwards. So incorporating a subjective probability will inevitably hurt the model.

On the other hand, the indirect factors like personality and background of the managers may be the actual influential factors in capital structure decision-making, or the factors lead to bias of capital structure decision, but are irrelevant to the optimal capital structure or rational capital structure decision, hence are not necessary to be incorporated into the model.

(6) Unlike the prevailing stochastic or other complex models, the ZZ leverage model is an explicit and analytical model, involves less mathematics and the calculation is easy by using the common software, such as Excel, etc.; there is no immeasurable variable like utility etc.; the independent variables are easy to estimate based on commonly accessible data. While the volatility (σ) may be not as easy as other variables to estimate, it is the most basic and most common measure of risk. Hence, the ZZ leverage model is totally feasible in terms of the understanding and application in practice. This feature is actual essential for a good financial model, since finance is a practice oriented science.

(7) Unlike the prevailing dynamic models, the ZZ leverage model is a simple and static model. Dynamic model, though fashionable in current academic research, is infeasible in practice, because it is neither possible nor necessary for a firm to adjust its debt ratio continuously or dynamically. Since capital structure adjustment involves adjustment cost, most firms only want to adjust their debt ratios occasionally; and the best choice is adjusting when they need additional capital. As a firm raises capitals from round to round, it can adjust its capital structure towards the optimum again and again. For such a purpose, an effective and efficient static optimal capital structure model is enough.

All above features are obviously essential for the model to remain its properness across times and markets and for further theoretical research and practical application.

5.5.3 Basic Insights from the Model

The basic relationships revealed

The ZZ leverage model incorporates four conditional variables and reveals the relationships between the four variables and the optimal capital structure: the corporate tax rate (f), the risk free rate (r), the debt maturity (T) as well as the firm value volatility (σ).

Based on the ZZ leverage model, the optimal debt ratio is positive related with the tax rate and negative related with the volatility of the firm's value; these are obviously make sense and in line with the common intuition. The relationships of the four conditional variables to the optimal debt ratio revealed by the model are summarized in Table 5.1.

Table 5.1 The relationships between the conditional variables and the optimal debt ratio ("+" represents positive related, and "–" represents negative related)

Conditional variable	Denotation	Relation
Corporate income tax rate	f	+
Risk-free interest rate	r	+
Maturity of the debt	T	–
Volatility of the firm value	σ	–

5.5 Decision-Oriented Optimal Capital Structure Model

While some relationships revealed by the model are easy to understand, such as that between the optimal leverage and the corporate tax rate and the firm value volatility, some relationships in the model are not so easy to understand, such as that between the optimal leverage and the other two conditional variables (r and T).

Based on the ZZ leverage model, the optimal debt ratio is positive related with the risk free rate and negative related with the maturity of the debt. These seem somehow not consistent with the common intuition. The risk free rate determines various interest rates to a large extent. When the risk free rate and interest rate increase, firms are supposed to use less debt, so is it really possible that they lift their leverages in such a circumstance?

There is a possibility that the increase of the debt ratio and the decrease of the debt size coexist on the condition that the equity capital decreases more than the debt does. That is true when the interest rate increases. The interest rate increase represents the increase in the debt cost. In reality, the debt cost cannot increase alone without a concurrent increase in equity cost. The capital transfer in capital market will rebalance the cost relationship between debt and equity. Therefore, when the interest rate increases, the equity cost will increase as well. The increase of the equity cost will restrain the use of equity and result in the increase of the debt ratio. Thus, when the risk free rate increases, the less uses of debt and equity can decrease and increase the optimal debt ratio respectively. But what is the net effect of the two contrary movements? It seems hard for us to decide by intuition. Fortunately, the ZZ leverage model tells us that the net effect is increase in optimal debt ratio.

As for the variable of debt maturity T, a common reasoning is that long term debt is somehow more similar to equity, or is safer (from the issuers' point of view) than short term debt. The debt maturity and the optimal leverage ratio hence should be positively related to each other. Leland and Toft [15], Stohs and Mauer [16], among others, stand for this viewpoint. On the contrary, Dennis et al. (2000) show that leverage is inversely related to debt maturity by their regressions. They argue that this happens because agency costs may be limited by reducing leverage and shortening debt maturity.

It is actually not necessary to bother with agency cost to explain the relationship between the debt maturity and the optimal debt ratio, since the reasoning can be quite simple based on the ZZ leverage model. Uncertainty will increase with the increase of the debt maturity, which will increase the bankruptcy cost (cost from debt financing). The optimal debt ratio thus should decrease as the debt maturity increase. A fact in reality supports this reasoning, i.e. other things being equal it is easier to borrow more short term debt than long term debt.

The value-addition potential from optimizing the leverage

How much can financing or capital structure decision add value to a firm? This is one of the important questions that capital structure research tries but fails to answer. Traditionally, scholars expect a significant value-addition from capital structure, just as something shown in Fig. 5.1, which is usually appearing in finance textbooks.[11]

---

[11] Such as Ross et al. [17], Brealey and Myers [18].

Without a convincing optimal capital structure model, Fig. 5.1 is drawn based on subjective guess, which is inevitably too subjective. For instance, is the value-addition potential from optimizing the leverage really as large as that shown in Fig. 5.1?

Based on the ZZ tax shield model and the ZZ bankruptcy cost model, take the base case firm as an example, where, f = 30 %; r = 3.0 %; T = 4; σ = 26 %, a similar figure can be depicted as Fig. 5.3. Because the firm and its related variables are typical, and the ZZ tax shield model and ZZ bankruptcy cost model are all derived based on correct concepts and strict logics, the curves and their positions are objective and have practical meaning.

It is interesting and meaningful to make a comparison between Figs. 5.1 and 5.3. There are firm values with and without trade-off value in both figures. In both figures, the curve of firm value with trade-off value (levered firm value) is rising first and falling then; and the curve of firm value without trade-off value (unlevered firm value) is level.

However, there is significant difference between Figs. 5.1 and 5.3. The curve of levered firm value in Fig. 5.1 is much higher over the curve of unlevered firm value, which implies that the trade-off value is an important part in the levered firm; whereas the curve of levered firm value in Fig. 5.3 is just slightly higher over the curve of unlevered firm value at around the optimal leverage, which implies that the trade-off value is not an significant part of the levered firm value, or the potential value-addition from capital structure decision is limited or insignificant.

In addition, according to Fig. 5.3, comparing with optimal leverage, the cost of over-leverage is asymmetrically higher than the cost of under-leverage. When debt ratio is relatively low, the firm value increases along with the increasing of debt ratio, but the potential value-addition is limited. Take the base case firm as an example, where f = 30 %, r = 3.0 %, T = 4, σ = 26 %, the optimal leverage ratio L = 33.80 %. This means that when the firm has unlevered value S = 100, the optimal size (value) of the debt X = 33.80. At this point,

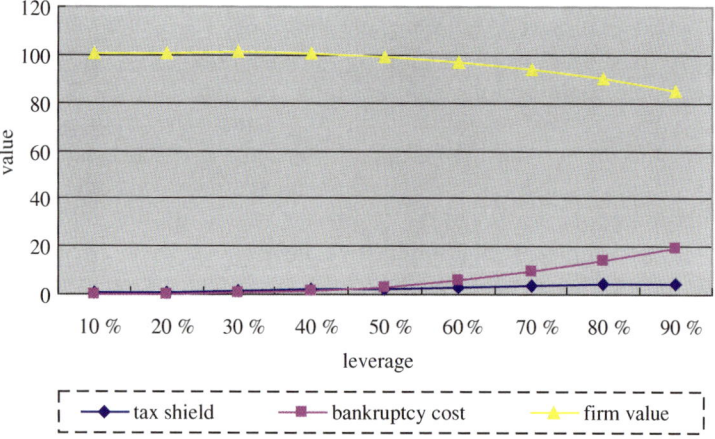

Fig. 5.3 The tax shield, bankruptcy cost and firm value

The tax shield = $Xf(1 - e^{-rT}) = 33.8030\% \times (1 - e^{-3.0\% \times 4}) = 1.15$
The bankruptcy cost = $XN(-d2) - SN(-d1) = 0.20$

This firm (a typical firm) will get value-addition of 0.95 (= 1.15 − 0.20) or less than 1 % of the original firm value 100 at most via the continuously optimal usage of debt capital until the debt maturity. In reality, no firm can keep its leverage on optimum during any year because the value of its equity fluctuates endlessly in the market, needless to say during the whole debt life. Thus the value-addition from capital structure decision is much lower than what widely expected or guessed so far. On the other hand, over-leverage will damage much of the firm value. For instance, if the typical firm uses more debt and reaches a leverage ratio of 51.5 %, the tax shield (1.75) is just canceled out by the bankruptcy cost (1.75); the trade off value is zero; the levered firm cannot obtain any value-addition from the usage of debt. If leverage ratio of the typical firm reaches 90 %, the tax shield is 3.05; the bankruptcy cost is 14.88; the trade off value is −11.82; the levered firm gets a negative value-addition so that the firm value decreases from 100 to 88.18, or decreases by 11.82 %.

5.5.4 Assumptions of the Model

As mentioned above, to obtain a basic theoretical and practical solution, we follow relative simple assumptions, thus solve the optimal capital structure with least number of variables which can meet the most important requirements and features of the relevant practical decision. Nevertheless, understanding the differences between these assumptions and the reality are helpful for various applications of the optimal leverage model.

The main assumptions under the ZZ leverage model include:

A. All debts are loans or bonds on credit; there is no guaranteed debt.
B. No transaction cost for both equity financing and debt financing; hence no adjustment cost for firms to change their capital structures.
C. No personal income tax on personal income from debt or equity investment.
D. The firm value grows compounding-continuously at risk free rate; no abnormal return or growth during the debt life.
E. No inter-firm investments, in other words, no part of a firm's assets functioning concurrently as the support of other firm's debt obligation.
F. The debt is fair-priced so that we can value the tax shield by discounting the annual tax savings at b, hence cancel the variable of b in the derivation process.
G. As assumed in the Black–Scholes option pricing model, the firm value moves similarly as its equity, i.e., follows a geometric Brownian motion (GBM) with a constant volatility σ so that we can apply the option pricing model.

The assumptions A, B, C, D, E and F may be somehow different from the reality. For instance, the guaranteed or mortgage debts are common in reality; there are indeed transaction costs for both equity financing and debt financing; there may be indeed taxes on personal income from debt investment and equity investment; firms may grow faster or slower than the risk free rate or even expected to grow negatively in the future; there are indeed inter-firm investments, such as receivables and various equity investments; the debt may be more or less mispriced because of various reasons; etc. We try to relax these assumptions and find the relevant special solutions in next section.

As for assumption G, although the firm value may move away from GBM sometime in reality due to special events, GBM is still a reasonable approximation of firm value dynamics except for rare events; and it is also among the simplest of stochastic processes. Within reasonable range, we should prefer simplicity to accuracy, because simplicity is a rare advantage for theoretical solutions and practical decisions. No models can be based on assumptions completely in line with the reality. Models on simple assumptions give more efficiencies and flexibilities for applications as long as the assumptions are roughly realistic.

There are also other assumptions implied in our model, such as that the business activities of a firm are unchanged by its capital structure, that the bankruptcy is only possible at the debt maturity when the firm value less than its debt full value (Xe^{rT}), etc. In reality, the firm activities may be changed more or less by its capital structure, but it is not commonly important. Similarly, a firm may go to bankrupt before or after its debt maturity, or the bankruptcy threshold may be somehow higher or lower than its debt value on maturity; but these cases are no longer difficult to solve with the ZZ model series on leverage.

Financial issues in reality are complex; no model can take all assumptions and factors into account. Assumptions behind a financial model different from reality can make an endless list, such as constant volatility, constant risk free rate, no dividends, perfect capital market, etc. Nevertheless, for the simplicity, feasibility, efficiency and flexibility of the model, we will not consider further the less important factors or the indirect factors. As mentioned earlier, most of the indirect factors have been incorporated already into the four independent variables of the ZZ model series on leverage.

5.6 Some Application Extensions

As theoretical models, the ZZ leverage related models have clear logic bases, hence is not difficult to extend for incorporating further some additional assumptions and variables. We intend to explore the applications of the ZZ leverage related models in various special situations in this section by relaxing some of the assumptions mentioned in last section and account for more common special factors in actual capital structure decisions.

5.6.1 Abnormal Growth

We have already accounted for firm value growth at a risk-free rate in the ZZ leverage model by applying the option pricing model. A firm may grow faster or slower during its debt life in reality. Suppose a firm is expected to grow at an

5.6 Some Application Extensions

abnormal rate of g in addition to r. How should we account for the additional growth rate of g?

Firm value S is the present value of its value at the debt maturity, S_T. In absence of abnormal growth, $S_T = Se^{rT}$; the firm value now is $S = Se^{rT}e^{-rT}$. If the firm's debt X reaches its optimum now, the firm reaches its optimal leverage ratio $L = X/S$. Other things being equal, when the values of the firm and its debt grow normally, the optimal leverage ratio at the debt maturity is the same as now, i.e., $L = (Xe^{rT})/(Se^{rT}) = X/S$.

With the abnormal growth at g in addition to r, the firm values now and on debt maturity are Se^{gT} and $Se^{rT}e^{gT}$ respectively. Suppose the debt value is not affected by the firm value's growth, or it remains growing at a risk-free rate and to be Xe^{rT} on the maturity. The debt ratio at debt maturity is: $(Xe^{rT})/(Se^{rT}e^{gT})$. This implies that to reach the optimal leverage X/S at the debt maturity, the leverage ratio now should be:

$$\begin{aligned} L = X/S &= \left(Xe^{rT}\right)/\left(Se^{rT}e^{gT}\right) \times e^{gT} \\ &= e^{gT + probit(f - fe^{-rT})\sigma\sqrt{T} - \sigma^2 T/2} \\ &= \exp\left\{gT + \left[probit\left(f - fe^{-rT}\right)\right]\sigma\sqrt{T} - \sigma^2 T/2\right\} \end{aligned} \quad (5.19)$$

As an example, assume the same values of f, r, σ, T as in the base case, except that the firm has an abnormal growth rate $g = 15.0$ % (so that the total growth rate is 18.0 %). Suppose that the firm intends to reach optimal leverage at the debt maturity, i.e. $X/(Se^{gT}) = 33.80$ %; thus the optimal debt ratio now should be: 33.80 % $\times e^{15\% \times 4} = 61.59$ %.

Note that the above reasoning can be applied to satisfy any growth pattern as well as any leverage policy of the firm. If the firm is expected to grow abnormally at 15 % during only 2 years, or the firm intends to reach an optimal leverage in the end of year 2 for some reasons, the optimal leverage now is 33.80 % $\times e^{15\% \times 2} = 45.62$ %.

It is commonly believed that firms with high return on total assets (ROA) should use more debt capital and have high leverages, because debt financing can increase share holders' return (ROE, return on equity) in such cases. The above analyses confirm this common sense. As illustrated in above analyses, the higher the growth rate, the higher the optimal leverage ratio. Since high growth rates are usually resulted from high return[12] (ROA), hence the higher the ROA, the higher the optimal leverage ratio.

5.6.2 Bankruptcy Expectancy

Bankruptcy expectancy implies the firm grows negatively during the debt life. We can account for such bankruptcy expectancy similarly as the "abnormal growth", except that the growth rate will be negative rather than positive.

---

[12] Growth rate is determined by the rate of return of the firm's investment and its dividend policy. Given the dividend policy, the growth rate is positively related to the rate of return.

Suppose the base case firm value is originally 100, and its debt value is originally 33.8. Now the firm value is expected to be 20 (<33.8) at the debt maturity, hence the firm will go bankrupt then. The annual growth rate during the debt life is $\sqrt[4]{20/100} - 1 = -33.13\ \%$. Assume the same inputs as the base case firm except that the firm has a total growth rate $-33.13\ \%$ (so that the abnormal growth rate is $g = -33.13\ \% - 3.0\ \% = -36.13\ \%$). Hence the optimal capital structure now is: $33.80\ \% \times e^{-36.13\ \% \times 4} = 7.97\ \%$.

The optimal leverage ratio decreases sharply comparing to the original level of 33.80 %. Actually, the bankruptcy expectancy may even drive the optimal leverage ratio down to zero. When a firm moves towards bankruptcy, it normally suffers from continuous loss without hope to recover to be profitable. Thus it has little chance to carry the loss forwards and to benefit from the tax shield of the debt capital. The debt can only contribute bankruptcy cost to the firm in such a case. This justifies an optimal leverage ratio of 0 %.

Hence firms with bankruptcy expectancy can hardly borrow in reality. However, firms before bankruptcy may have high debt ratios. This just reflects that the ex-bankruptcy or distressed firms postpone their repaying of the due debts and their firm value decline sharply. The relatively high debt ratios are by no means the optimal leverages in such a case. This reminds us that an optimal leverage model cannot be derived from or to justified by sample data. In other words, theoretical research (based on correct concepts and strict logic) is the only possible way to solve the problem of optimal capital structure.

5.6.3 Market Value Versus Book Value

Some surveys reveal that firms are concerned more on book values.[13] Following the financial research convention, the ZZ leverage related models are on market value basis, but it is not difficult to translate the market value leverage into its corresponding book value leverage.

The market value of debt is usually close to its book value as long as the firm keeps healthy, so the debt market/book ratio is usually close to 1. The market value of equity may be several times of its book value. The equity market value of a publicly traded firm is the product of its share price and number of shares outstanding. The equity market value of a privately held firm can be determined according to the similar publicly traded firms. Therefore, it is possible to estimate the equity market/book ratio of a firm.

For the base case firm, assume the market/book ratio of equity is 4; the market/book ratio of debt is 1; and current book debt ratio is 60 % or book equity ratio is 40 %. The market/book ratio of the firm then is $(4 \times 40\ \% + 1 \times 60\ \%)/(1 \times 40\ \% + 1 \times 60\ \%) = 2.2$, or the firm market value equal its book value

---

[13] Such as Servaes and Tufano [19].

multiplied by 2.2. As the optimal leverage ratio L (=X/S) at market value is 33.80 %, the optimal leverage ratio L at book value is 33.80 % × 2.2 = 74.36 %.

For the convenience in expression, hereafter, we refer to debt or leverage ratio on book value as book debt or leverage ratio, and debt or leverage ratio on market value as market debt or leverage ratio. Note that the 74.36 % is different from the original book debt ratio 60 %, which is an input to derive the result of 74.36 %. This implies some interactions between the original book debt ratio and the derived optimal book debt ratio. So we can use the "goal seek" of Excel to find the optimal book leverage ratio. The final result is 67.13 %.

The result can be checked this way: the book equity ratio is: 1 − 67.13 % = 32.87 %. Thus, the market debt ratio is: 67.13 %/(67.13 % + 4 × 32.87 %) = 33.80 %. This illustrates that the optimal book debt ratio of 67.13 % is equivalent to the optimal market debt ratio of 33.80 %. To generalize the above process, denote the optimal book leverage by L′, the market/book ratio of the equity by m, the optimal market leverage ratio is:

$$L = \frac{L'}{L' + m(1-L')} \quad (5.20)$$

Thus, the model of optimal book leverage ratio is:

$$L' = \frac{m}{1/L + m - 1} \quad (5.21)$$

Where L is determined by Eqs. 5.15 or 5.18, and the market/book ratio of debt is assumed to be 1. Thus, we can find the optimal book leverage ratio based on Eqs. 5.15 or 5.18 and 5.21. Clearly, when m = 1 in Eq. 5.21, L′ = L.

5.6.4 Guaranteed Debt

Guaranteed debts are even more common than credit debts in reality, especially for small firms. When a firm has debt guaranteed by an outside or independent guarantor, it has to pay for the guarantee. Previous research reveals that the fair guarantee fee equals to a put option value which is just as the same one used to hedge the bankruptcy risk in Sect. 5.4.3. So, the bankruptcy cost of the guaranteed debt doubles (200 %) that of the credit debt. Based on Eq. 5.15, for a guaranteed debt, the optimal leverage satisfies:

$$2N[\frac{\ln(L)}{\sigma\sqrt{T}} + \frac{\sigma\sqrt{T}}{2}] = f(1 - e^{-rT}) \quad (5.22)$$

Similarly, Eq. 5.18 should be rewritten as:

$$L = e^{probit(f/2 - fe^{-rT}/2)\sigma\sqrt{T} - \sigma^2 T/2}$$
$$= \exp\left\{[probit(f/2 - fe^{-rT}/2)]\sigma\sqrt{T} - \sigma^2 T/2\right\} \quad (5.23)$$

According to Eqs. 5.22 or 5.23, the effect of debt guarantee on the optimal capital structure is equivalent to that of a half reduction of the corporate tax rate.

Take the base case firm again as an example, other things being equal, i.e. $f = 30\ \%$, $r = 3.0\ \%$, $T = 4$, $\sigma = 26\ \%$, but the firm needs a guarantee for its debt and pays a fair upfront guarantee fee. Based on Eqs. 5.22 or 5.23, the optimal leverage now is 28.99 %, which is lower than the original optimal leverage of 33.80 %. This reflects the guarantee makes the debt financing less attractive. Why some small firms or startups with high growth rates have lower leverage ratios? Why are they likely to use equity capital? Now we know one reason is that they have to find debt guarantees for their debt financing; the difficulties and the additional costs from debt guarantees make the debt financing less attractive.

5.6.5 Transaction Costs

There are normally transaction costs associated with financing. When firms issue bonds, there are underwriting spreads as well as registration and legal fees. When firms borrow from banks, there may be also some implicit or explicit costs in addition to the interest costs. Similarly, when firms raise funds with equity, there are also or even more substantial transaction costs as a fraction of the amount of the capital raised.

In case of the transaction costs, firms had better to adjust their capital structures by the chance of financing, so that the adjustments will not generate additional transaction costs. On the other hand, a firm's capital structure will change automatically along with the fluctuations of its market value. This implies that it is not possible for a firm to keep on optimal leverage via continuous or dynamic adjustment. That is to say, a firm has to let its capital structure less optimal in between the adjustments or financing rounds. Leary and Roberts [20] show that the adjustment costs having a persistent effect on leverage.

While the transaction cost and adjustment cost are usually conceived as the same, in the context of capital structure decision, they are actually different in terms of the concepts and amount. The adjustment cost is the additional transaction cost for the capital structure adjustment. When a firm changes its capital structure by the chance of financing, it generates transaction cost but does not necessarily involve adjustment cost. Firms adjust their capital structure only when the adjustment benefits are large than the adjustment costs. What we should care about is the adjustment cost rather than the transaction cost.

Firms can adjust their capital structures by issuing debt or equity at financing. The transaction costs of debt or equity or both are necessary in despite of their capital structure adjustments. The adjustment cost as an additional cost is insignificant in such a case. However, when firms adjust their capital structures between two financing rounds, they need to issue additional equity and prepay some debt, or issue additional debt and repurchase some outstanding equity. In either case, the adjustment cost is the sum of the two-way transaction costs of debt and equity financing which is obviously significant.

Firms thus should adjust their capital structures by the chance of financing, so that they can avoid most of the adjustment costs. Under such a consideration, viewing from the debt side, the adjustment cost is the additional transaction cost of debt over equity financing, which can be either positive or negative. The additional debt transaction cost results from similar reasons as that of the guarantee fee, such as the uncertainty of the business or the insecurity of the debt repayment, and has the same features, such as both are the upfront payments. Thus, the adjustment costs can be treated in a similar way as that of the guarantee fee.

Suppose the expected adjustment cost of the debt financing sums to h times the guarantee fee, the ZZ leverage model should be rewritten as:

$$(1+h) N[\frac{\ln(L)}{\sigma\sqrt{T}} + \frac{\sigma\sqrt{T}}{2}] = f(1 - e^{-rT}) \tag{5.24}$$

Or,

$$\begin{aligned} L &= e^{probit[1-f(e^{-rT})/(1+h)]\sigma\sqrt{T}-\sigma^2 T/2} \\ &= \exp\{[probit(f - fe^{-rT})/(1+h)]\sigma\sqrt{T} - \sigma^2 T/2\} \end{aligned} \tag{5.25}$$

According to Eqs. 5.24 or 5.25, the effect of an adjustment cost of the debt financing on the capital structure decision is equivalent to replacing the corporate tax rate f by f/(1 + h). Exemplifying again with the base case firm, assume the same values for f, r, σ and T, except that the firm now needs to pay an additional upfront transaction cost (adjustment cost) proportional as 30 % of the debt guarantee fee. Based on Eqs. 5.24 or 5.25, the optimal capital structure is now 31.83 %.

The adjustment cost makes the debt financing slightly less attractive. Of course, if the debt is cheaper than equity in terms of transaction cost, it will be more attractive. For instance, other things being equal, but comparing with the equity financing, the debt financing has a negative additional transaction cost totaling up to −30 % of the guarantee fee. Based on Eqs. 5.24 or 5.25, the optimal leverage ratio is 36.85 %. Thus, the transaction cost advantage makes the debt financing slightly more attractive.

5.6.6 Personal Income Tax

As the same reasoning of the transaction cost, for the capital structure decision, the personal income tax is only relevant when there is significant difference in personal income tax between debt income and equity income. Anyway, we can extend the ZZ leverage model to incorporate this factor whenever it is necessary.

The debt interest as personal income is usually taxed at a higher rate than the income from the stock, which results in a "personal tax penalty" related to the interest payments. Therefore, investors usually demand a higher pre-tax return for their debt capitals. Thanks to Miller's contribution (Miller's formula [21]), we can account for the "personal tax penalty" by using $[1 - \frac{(1-f)(1-f_{pe})}{(1-f_{pd})}]$ to replace f in the ZZ leverage model.

$$N[\frac{\ln(L)}{\sigma\sqrt{T}} + \frac{\sigma\sqrt{T}}{2}] = [1 - \frac{(1-f)(1-f_{pe})}{(1-f_{pd})}](1 - e^{-rT}) \quad (5.26)$$

Or,

$$L = e^{\{probit[1 - \frac{(1-f)(1-f_{pe})}{(1-f_{pd})}](1-e^{-rT})\}\,\sigma\sqrt{T} - \sigma^2 T/2}$$

$$= \exp\{[probit \frac{(1-f_{pd})(1 - e^{-rT}) - (1-f)(1-f_{pe})(1 - e^{-rT})}{(1-f_{pd})}] \quad (5.27)$$

$$\times \sigma\sqrt{T} - \sigma^2 T/2\}$$

Where f is still the corporate tax rate, f_{pe} is the personal tax rate on income from equity investment, and f_{pd} is the personal tax rate on income from debt investment.

Again, take the base case firm as an example, other things being equal, i.e. f = 30 %, r = 3.0 %, T = 4, σ = 26 %, assume further f_{pe} = 10 %, f_{pd} = 20 %. Thus $[1 - \frac{(1-f)(1-f_{pe})}{(1-f_{pd})}] = 21.25$ %. Based on Eqs. 5.26 or 5.27, the optimal leverage ratio is L = 31.25 %.

Comparing with the original optimum 33.80 %, the personal tax penalty makes the debt financing slightly less attractive. Understandingly, if the personal tax rate on equity income exceeds that on debt income, i.e. a special situation with negative personal tax penalty, the debt financing will be more attractive. For instance, other things being equal, but f_{pd} = 0 %. Then $[1 - \frac{(1-f)(1-f_{pe})}{(1-f_{pd})}] = 37$ %. Based on Eqs. 5.26 or 5.27, the optimal leverage ratio is 35.53 %, which implies the debt financing is slightly more attractive.

5.6.7 Inter-Firm's Investments

Consider ten firms in an economy with firm value 100, 200, 300, ..., 1000 million dollars respectively. The total value of these firms is 5500 million dollars. If these firms are all the "typical" firms (like the base case firm), their optimal debts should be: 33.80 % × 100 = 33.80, 33.80 % × 200 = 67.60, 33.80 % × 300 = 101.40, ..., 33.80 % × 1000 = 338.0 million dollars respectively. The optimal debt ratio for the ten firms as a whole is 33.80 %, or the sum of the ten firms' optimal debt are 33.80 % × 5500 = 1859.0 million dollars.

However, firms in reality are not isolated. They have various relations with each other. A common relation is that they invest capital in or receive capital from other firms. The investments may take various forms, such as receivables (payables) or some long-term investments as debt or equity. Because of this, part of a firm's value may be also part of another firm's value. For instance, a firm's receivables may be just another firm's payables.

Therefore, the total value of the above ten firms is likely less than 5500 million dollars. If every firm has 30 % value as the investments (equity or/and debt) in other firms, the total assets of the ten firms, which can be used to support their debt repayments, is $(1 - 30\,\%) \times 5500 = 3850$ million dollars. Thus the total optimal debt of the ten firms is $33.80\,\% \times 3850 = 1301.3$ million dollars. This implies the average optimal debt ratio is 23.66 % ($= (1 - 30\,\%) \times 33.80\,\%$) rather than 33.80 % when all the firms are regarded as isolated to each others.

The capital structure in reality is not only the choice of the firm (debtor), but also the choice of the lender (creditor), such as the commercial banks. Lenders want their money safe, or they want every debt has enough assets at its back. Even the above ten firms prefer a capital structure of 33.80 % debt, lenders who are rational enough to know the inter-firm's investment may insist that the debt ratio of every firm is not obviously more than 23.66 %.

The applications above illustrated that the ZZ model series on leverage is flexible enough to accommodate capital structure decisions in various real situations.

5.7 Explanations to Some Capital Structure Puzzles

Since the problem of optimal capital structure have remained unsolved for decades, more and more empirical observations are found inconsistent with academic hypotheses, which are referred to as capital structure puzzles. We explore some of them and provide alternative explanations in this section based on the ZZ leverage model.

5.7.1 Why Financial Conservatism

Based on overvalued tax shields and undervalued bankruptcy costs, prior studies assume subjectively higher optimal leverage ratios. Consequently, the leverage ratios in reality seem too low. Graham (2000, 22) finds that conservative debt policy (under-levered financing) is a persistent and pervasive capital structure puzzle. According to Tserlukevich [23], the optimal market leverage ratio generally falls between 43 and 73 %; while the common market leverage ratios reported by various surveys lie between 29 and 35 %.

Financial scholars create a terminology of "financial conservatism" to bridge the gap between the academic hypotheses and the reality, which implies that firms are too conservative in borrowing. However, the optimal leverage ratio 33.80 % derived based on the ZZ leverage model is close to many survey results. Thus a more convincing explanation may be: the "theoretical standards" are too radical, and the actual leverage ratios are roughly appropriate. According to last section, the inter-firm investments will drive the optimal debt ratios even lower. Therefore, firms on average behave properly rather than conservatively.

As what we find in last section, for a typical firm, where f = 30 %, r = 3.0 %, T = 4, σ = 26 %, the optimal leverage ratio L = 33.80 %, and the value-addition resulted from the optimal usage of debt capital is very limited (only 0.95 of the firm value). In addition, as revealed in "Sect. 5.5.3", the cost of being overlevered is asymmetrically higher than the cost of being underlevered. For instance, if the typical firm reaches a leverage ratio of 90 %, the firm value decreases by 11.82 %. Under-leverage will not hurt the firm value much; but over-leverage will led to a big loss of the firm value.

Why so many firms behave conservatively in financing? Now the reason cannot be clearer. Firms do not know how to find a precise optimal leverage, but they sense intuitively that over leverage may damage their firms' value seriously. In such a case, the lower or even zero debt ratios are all rational choices in absence of a reliable optimal leverage model, because it is not worthy to risk a big loss for a very limited value addition.

5.7.2 Why No Leverage Target

Prior research documents that many firms have no leverage target.[14] Now, based on the ZZ leverage model, we can explain this phenomenon as follows.

Firstly, there has been no reliable model with theoretical soundness and practical feasibility to support actual capital structure decisions, but practitioners sense that the potential of the value-addition via debt financing is very limited, so it is not worthy to spend much management times and efforts on determining and maintaining a "leverage target".

Secondly, there are various constrains for many firms to raise their necessary capitals in reality. Thus firms may just choose the most convenient way to raise their capitals. They do not care the capitals are equity or debt, or the effect of their choice on their capital structures, so long as their debts do not bring in too much bankruptcy risk.

Thirdly, because both debt and equity financing have transaction costs, adjusting capital structures will involve adjustment costs. Firms prefer to only adjust their capital structures by the chance of financing and let the debt ratios drift between financings, regardless how far of their capital structures from the leverage targets (if they have the targets).

A firm may reach its optimal capital structure at a debt/equity issuance. Then the firm value changes inevitably with its business performance and the capital market conditions. This implies the debt ratios of most firms deviate from optimums most of the time. Thus, researchers actually cannot find leverage targets for most firms based on sample data.

---

[14] See among others, Bradley et al. [24], Graham and Harvey [22].

5.7.3 Why Averse-Change With Profitability

Theoretically, firms can use more debt financing when they are expected to get more profitable. However, some scholars find significant exceptions, i.e., the leverage ratio decreases as the profitability increases, such as Strebulaev [25].

When firms decide on whether or not to adjust capital structures, they should trade-off between the adjustment cost and the value-addition from the adjustment. Based on the above discussions, as the value-addition from adjusting capital structure is very limited, firms usually do not change their debt size before the next financing.

However, if a firm gets more profitable, its value will increase immediately in the market and its debt ratio will consequently decrease. Therefore, an increase in profitability "naturally" lowers leverage by increasing future profits and the current firm value. As the same reasoning, a decrease in profitability "naturally" reduces firm value and raises leverage.

In short, because firms only adjust their capital structures periodically, their debt ratios drift naturally in a way of averse-changes with profitability most of the time.

5.7.4 Why Over Stable Leverage

Some scholars find that some firms do not adjust their capital structure in time even when some important conditions change significantly,[15] such as the changes of the corporate tax rate and the risk free rate. Now we can explain this phenomenon as follows.

Firstly, there has been no decision-oriented model to determine the debt ratio; firms do not know how much debt they should add or reduce to reach the optimum after the relevant conditions change. To avoid unnecessary risk, they just copy their past experiences, and maintain their capital structures even they have adjusting opportunities.

Secondly, based on the ZZ leverage model, the optimal debt ratio is not very sensitive to some conditions, such as the corporate tax rate, the risk free rate, etc., although they are important conditional variables for capital structure decisions.

For instance, other things being equal in the base case firm, but the corporate tax rate changes from 30 to 40 %, based on the ZZ leverage model, the optimal debt ratio will change to 36.22 %, which is not far from the original 33.80 %. Based on the ZZ trade off value, if the leverage maintained at 33.80 % (which is no longer the optimum), the firm value is 101.33; if the leverage is adjusted to the new optimum of 36.22 %, the firm value is 101.35. The firm value increases by 0.02 % at most through the leverage adjustment. Obviously, the leverage adjustment makes no sense even in absence of adjustment cost.

---

[15] See among others, Mackie-Mason and Jeffrey (1990), Fama and French (2002).

The analysis above can also explain why firms seem to have optimal leverage ranges rather than precise optimal leverage targets. We thus conclude: theoretically, there is indeed a precise optimal leverage for every firm at a certain time; but practically, a firm needs to rebalance its leverage only when it drifts far away from the optimum.

5.7.5 Why Pecking Order

Myers and Majluf 26 suggest that firms follow financing priorities to minimize information asymmetry between the firm's insiders (managers) and the outsiders (shareholders), i.e., they prefer internal sourced capitals like depreciation funds, retained earnings, etc. to outside sourced capitals; when they have to raise outside sourced capitals, they prefer debt to equity. This is referred to as pecking order hypothesis or pecking order theory.

Based on what we find so far, as the potential value-addition from the leverage adjustment is very limited, the leverage decision is not as important as other management decisions for a firm to pursue its value-maximization target, such as investment and operating decisions. Therefore, firms are more likely to choose a convenient way to raise their capital, so long as the debt capital is not much as a fraction of their total capital.

For most firms, the internal sourced capitals are the most convenient capitals. So, those internal sourced capitals are often the first ordered capitals. Beyond those capitals, however, there should be no certain pecking order for most firms. Firms in different environment have different favorite pecking order. For instance, while some researchers find that firms prefer debt to equity, publicly listed firms in China prefer equity to debt. There is actually no certain or unified pecking order for firms across markets and periods; firms simply choose their pecking order according to the ever-changing internal and external conditions.

There may be a pecking order for every firm over a certain period to financing its business, but the reason behind this order is not as complicated as guessed in prevailing research literature, such as information asymmetry, etc. It is just because every firm has its own advantage over various financing channels, so it may choose equity or debt first. Besides, the information asymmetry is not likely to be the consideration of top importance in firms' decision. The ultimate target for most firms is maximizing its value which should be the first ordered consideration in financing as well as capital structure decisions. If reducing information asymmetry outweighs maximizing firm value, firms should not do any business; they should just sell all the assets and deposit all the proceeds in banks.

In addition, the pecking order hypothesis actually cannot eliminate the problem of optimal capital structure. Suppose firms really make financing decision based on their "pecking order", there is still a problem of "what is the best debt ratio at which they should turn to the second ordered capital". More importantly, while most scholars regard the pecking order hypothesis as contrary to the optimal capital structure, it is actually not. Financing convenience may outweigh optimizing capital structure in some circumstances. That firms have pecking order for financing does not necessarily mean that they have no optimal capital structure.

In academic area, every issue is regarded as most important in the relevant field; but in practice, the importance varies a lot across managerial decisions. Firms make the important decisions carefully and make the less important decisions at their convenience. Firms may sense that there is an optimal leverage, but they just do not care, because optimizing capital structure is not as beneficial as regarded by scholars.

5.7.6 Why Market Timing

Some scholars find that the equity market timing is an influential factor on firms' capital structures, such as Graham and Harvey [22], Baker and Wurgler [27], Ilch (2004), etc. They suggest that firms issue new shares when their shares are overvalued and repurchase outstanding shares when their shares are undervalued. Consequently, fluctuations in stock prices affect firm's capital structures, and the current capital structure is the cumulative outcome of past attempts to time the equity market.

Many scholars regard the market timing theory or hypothesis as a contrary to the optimal capital structure (trade-off theory). This is a misunderstanding similar to the relation between the optimal capital structure and the pecking order hypothesis. The ZZ leverage model reveals that the pure capital structure consideration is not as important as other managerial or financial decisions, so it has less priority in firms' decision lists.

As analyzed above, for a typical firm, even it keeps continuously on optimal leverage during the debt life, the potential value-addition at most is 0.95 %. However, the issuing price of stock may vary far beyond 10 % at different time. Therefore, it is a rational choice for a firm to make more efforts on (equity) market timing rather than capital structure, although there is indeed an optimal leverage ratio in theory.

Please note this is by no means that the market timing is a factor considered in capital structure decision; rather, the market timing and the capital structure are two competing decisions with different priorities. If you cannot give enough consideration to both, you have to ensure the market timing first. In other words, your capital structure may deviate from its optimum because of your market timing decision.

Obviously, while the market timing hypothesis may explain some actual capital structures (not necessarily optimal capital structure) to some extent, it cannot offer any help for solving the problem of optimal capital structure.

5.7.7 Dynamic Consideration?

In order to better explain the capital structures in reality, some scholars try to find insights beyond one single-period, such as Kane et al. [5] and Brennan and Schwartz [28], etc. Their arguments are referred to as the dynamic trade-off theory. Dynamic trade-off models also try to consider the option values embedded in deferring leverage decisions to the next period, such as Fischer et al. [29], Goldstein et al. [30] and Strebulaev [25].

In the dynamic models or hypothesis, a firm's leverage responds less to short-run equity fluctuations and more to long-run value changes. The optimal financial leverage choice today depends on what is expected to be optimal in the next period. Thus, the dynamic trade-off theory explains the chaotic actual leverages this way: although they seem not to be optimal in current period, they are expected to be optimal in next period.

Appearing brilliant with the "dynamic" label, the dynamic hypothesis is actually too academic. Firms may seem respond less to short-run fluctuations and more to long-run changes in their leverage decisions. However, this is not because they care their capital structure so much that they make a foresighted decision, but that they do not very care their capital structure so they only rebalance their leverage inactively.

Similar to the dynamic hypothesis, some scholars try to explain various capital structures puzzles by resorting to more factors far from tax shield and bankruptcy risk (cost), such as various macroeconomic factors, investment decision factors, and so on. Unfortunately, comparing with other important issues, it is not necessary for firms to care their capital structure so much; and they actually do not consider so much in their capital structure decisions. In other words, in absence of capital structure decision, they may still need to consider those macro or micro factors for the value creation of the firm.

5.7.8 Why Not 0 % Debt in Absence of Corporate Tax

A fact seems contradictory to the trade off between tax shield and bankruptcy cost in capital structure decision. Some scholars find that firms during early years in American had some debt in their capital mix even when there is no corporate income tax.

In the environment without corporate tax, firms financing with debt cannot obtain any tax shield. If they made their capital structure decision based on trading off between the benefits and cost of the debt financing, the final decision should be 0 % debt, because there is only cost from debt financing. But this is not the fact which seems hard to explain.

The fact is actually not contradictory at all to the trade off theory. The basic idea of the trade off theory is: other things being equal, a firm should trade off between tax shield and bankruptcy cost to make its capital structure decision. The "other things" include of course the firm's business. A firm often needs a certain amount of capital before a deadline for a business opportunity. The debt capital is often much more convenient to obtain than the equity capital; the firm is likely to miss the business opportunity without the debt financing. So it is natural for a firm to take the business opportunity by debt financing.

In such a case, the firm should give priority to the trade off between the benefit and cost of the business opportunity rather than between the tax shield and bankruptcy cost. In another words, the consideration on new investment is more important than that on financing. Just as what revealed by the ZZ leverage related models, the net benefit of the new business is likely much larger than the net benefit (cost) of debt financing over equity financing. That is why firms still use debt capital even when there is no corporate income tax and debt financing has net cost rather than net benefit. Anyway, the ZZ leverage model reveals also that too much debt may damage the firm value significantly. So, if it is too urgent to raise additional equity capital and the net benefit of the new business cannot cancel out the net cost of debt financing, the firm should give up the business opportunity.

Therefore, the fact that firms had some debt in their capital mix even when there is no corporate income tax is just the evidence that the value addition from leverage decision is not so important and the insights from the ZZ leverage related models are correct.

5.8 Summary

Optimal capital structure has been a bad headache in financial community. In front of the research difficulties and the impact of the empirical research "fashion", the relevant studies actually deviate from how to find the optimal capital structure to how to explain the existing capital structure (disregard it is optimal capital structure or not) in recent decades.

Unfortunately, the very limited efforts left to the real research on "optimal capital structure" are mostly based on the wrong concepts of tax shield and bankruptcy cost—the two most important concepts in optimal capital structure studies. That is why the problem of optimal capital structure remains unsolved after intensive studies of half century.

In this chapter, we revise the prior erroneous concepts and redefine the tax shield and bankruptcy cost on one round financing basis. Based on the correct concepts of tax shield and bankruptcy cost as well as the MM models and Black–Scholes model, we develop the ZZ model series on leverage, which include the ZZ tax shield model and the ZZ bankruptcy cost model as well as the ZZ optimal leverage condition and the ZZ leverage model.

The ZZ leverage (capital structure) model accounts basically for four variables to determine the optimal debt ratio, namely corporate income tax rate, risk-free interest rate, maturity of the debt and volatility of the firm value. Based on the typical values of the conditional variables, the optimal debt ratio (33.80 %) derived by the ZZ leverage model is significantly lower than the currently widespread "theoretical" standard (50 % or more). Therefore, it is straightforward to explain the long-lasting puzzle of "financial conservatism".

In addition, the ZZ model series on leverage can be easily extended to accommodate various decision situations and more conditional factors, such as abnormal growth, bankrupt expectancy, debt guarantee, transaction cost, personal income tax, etc. and can as well be used to explain better most of the other long-lasting capital structure puzzles. This implies that the ZZ model series on leverage are the effective and efficient solution.

Appendix

The Derivation of the Condition of Optimal Capital Structure

The condition of the optimal capital structure is that the ZZ trade-off value or the net benefit of the debt financing is maximized.

In the ZZ trade-off value model (Eq. 5.13), for a certain firm at a certain moment, other independent variables are given, and the X is the only variable for capital structure decision. Hence the condition of the optimal capital structure is equivalent to that the derivative of Eq. 5.13 with respect to X equals zero. To avoid the confusion of derivative operator "d" and the "d" in option pricing model and the ZZ leverage related models, I'd like to use an apostrophe (') to denote the derivative with respect to X in this Appendix.

ZZ Trade − off value $F(X) = fX(1 - e^{-rT}) - [XN(-d2) - SN(-d1)]$

Where $0 < X < S$

Let $F'(X) = 0$, i.e

$$\{fX(1 - e^{-rT}) - [XN(-d2) - SN(-d1)]\}' = 0 \quad (5.28)$$

$$\begin{aligned}
\{fX(1 - e^{-rT}) &- [XN(-d2) - SN(-d1)]\}' \\
&= [fX(1 - e^{-rT})]' - [XN(-d2) - SN(-d1)]' \\
&= f(1 - e^{-rT}) - [XN(-d2)]' + [SN(-d1)]' \\
&= f(1 - e^{-rT}) - N(-d2) - X[N(-d2)]' + S[N(-d1)]'
\end{aligned} \quad (5.29)$$

$$\text{Since } [N(x)]' = \frac{1}{\sqrt{2\pi}} e^{-\frac{x^2}{2}}$$

$$[N(-d2)]' = \frac{1}{\sqrt{2\pi}} e^{-\frac{(-d2)^2}{2}} (-d2)' \quad (5.30)$$

Appendix

$$(-d2)' = \left[-\frac{\ln(S/X)}{\sigma\sqrt{T}} + \frac{\sigma\sqrt{T}}{2}\right]'$$

$$= -\frac{\ln'(S/X)}{\sigma\sqrt{T}} = -\frac{(X/S)(S/X)'}{\sigma\sqrt{T}} \quad (5.31)$$

$$= -\frac{-(1/X)}{\sigma\sqrt{T}} = \frac{1}{X\sigma\sqrt{T}}$$

Thus,

$$[N(-d2)]' = \frac{1}{X\sigma\sqrt{T}} \frac{1}{\sqrt{2\pi}} e^{-\frac{(d2)^2}{2}} \quad (5.32)$$

And,

$$X[N(-d2)]' = \frac{1}{\sqrt{2\pi}} e^{-\frac{(d2)^2}{2}} \frac{1}{\sigma\sqrt{T}} \quad (5.33)$$

Similarly,

$$[N(-d1)]' = \frac{1}{\sqrt{2\pi}} e^{-\frac{(d1)^2}{2}} (-d1)'$$

$$= [-\frac{\ln(S/X)}{\sigma\sqrt{T}} - \frac{\sigma\sqrt{T}}{2}]' \frac{1}{\sqrt{2\pi}} e^{-\frac{(d1)^2}{2}} \quad (5.34)$$

$$= \frac{1}{X\sigma\sqrt{T}} \frac{1}{\sqrt{2\pi}} e^{-\frac{(d1)^2}{2}}$$

As $d2 = d1 - \sigma\sqrt{T}$, or $d1 = d2 + \sigma\sqrt{T}$,

Then $(d1)^2 = (d2 + \sigma\sqrt{T})^2$

$$= (d2)^2 + 2(d2)\sigma\sqrt{T} + \sigma^2 T$$

$$= (d2)^2 + 2\left[\frac{\ln(s/x)}{\sigma\sqrt{T}} - \frac{\sigma\sqrt{T}}{2}\right]\sigma\sqrt{T} + \sigma^2 T \quad (5.35)$$

$$= (d2)^2 + 2\ln(S/X) - \sigma^2 T + \sigma^2 T$$

$$= (d2)^2 + 2\ln(S/X)$$

According to 5.35 and 5.34,

$$\begin{aligned}
[N(-d1)]' &= \frac{1}{X\sigma\sqrt{T}} \frac{1}{\sqrt{2\pi}} e^{-\frac{(d1)^2}{2}} \\
&= \frac{1}{X\sigma\sqrt{T}} \frac{1}{\sqrt{2\pi}} e^{-\frac{(d2)^2 + 2\ln(S/X)}{2}} \\
&= \frac{1}{X\sigma\sqrt{T}} \frac{1}{\sqrt{2\pi}} e^{-\frac{(d2)^2}{2}} e^{-\ln(S/X)} \\
&= \frac{1}{X\sigma\sqrt{T}} \frac{1}{\sqrt{2\pi}} e^{-\frac{(d2)^2}{2}} e^{\ln(X/S)} \\
&= \frac{1}{X\sigma\sqrt{T}} \frac{1}{\sqrt{2\pi}} e^{-\frac{(d2)^2}{2}} \frac{X}{S} \\
&= \frac{1}{S\sigma\sqrt{T}} \frac{1}{\sqrt{2\pi}} e^{-\frac{(d2)^2}{2}}
\end{aligned} \quad (5.36)$$

Thus,

$$S[N(-d1)]' = \frac{1}{\sqrt{2\pi}} e^{-\frac{(d2)^2}{2}} \frac{1}{\sigma\sqrt{T}} \quad (5.37)$$

Based on 5.33 and 5.37,

$$X[N(-d2)]' = S[N(-d1)]' \quad (5.38)$$

Based on 5.38 and 5.29,

$$\begin{aligned}
F'(X) &= f(1 - e^{-rT}) - N(-d2) - X[N(-d2)]' + S[N(-d1)]' \\
&= f(1 - e^{-rT}) - N(-d2)
\end{aligned} \quad (5.39)$$

Thus, the condition of optimal capital structure is simplified as:

$$\begin{aligned}
f(1 - e^{-rT}) - N(-d2) &= 0 \text{ or} \\
f(1 - e^{-rT}) &= N(-d2)
\end{aligned} \quad (5.40)$$

Further, to make sure when $f(1-e^{-rT}) = N(-d2)$ the ZZ trade-off value or net benefit of the debt financing is being maximized rather than being minimized, we need to prove the second derivative of F(X) is negative, i.e. $[F'(X)]' < 0$.

According to 5.39 and 5.32,

$$\begin{aligned}
[F'(X)]' &= [f(1 - e^{-rT}) - N(-d2)]' \\
&= [-N(-d2)]' \\
&= -\frac{1}{X\sigma\sqrt{T}} \frac{1}{\sqrt{2\pi}} e^{-\frac{(d2)^2}{2}}
\end{aligned} \quad (5.41)$$

Because $\frac{1}{X\sigma\sqrt{T}} > 0$, $\frac{1}{\sqrt{2\pi}} > 0$, $e^{-\frac{(d2)^2}{2}} > 0$

Therefore, $[F'(X)]' < 0$, i.e., when the $F'(X) = f(1 - e^{-rT}) - N(-d2) = 0$, the ZZ trade-off value $F(X)$ gets maximized. Thus, Eq. 5.40 (i.e. Eq. 5.14 in "Sect. 5.5.1") is the condition of optimal capital structure.

References

1. Modigliani F, Miller MH (1958) The cost of capital, corporation finance and the theory of investment. Am Econ Rev 48:261–297
2. Modigliani F, Miller MH (1963) Corporate income taxes and the cost of capital: a correction. Am Econ Rev 53:433–443
3. Kraus A, Litzenberger R (1973) A state-preference model of optimal financial leverage. J Financ 28:911–922
4. DeAngelo H, Masulis R (1980) Optimal Capital Structure under Corporate Taxation. J Financ Econ 8:5–29
5. Kane A, Marcus A, McDonald R (1984) How big is the tax advantage to debt? J Financ 39:841–853
6. Miles J, Ezzell J (1985) Reformulating the tax shield: a note. J Financ 1485–1492
7. Graham JR (2000) How big are the tax benefits of debt? J Financ 55:1901–1941
8. Cooper IA, Nyborg K (2006) The value of tax shields IS equal to the present value of tax shields. J Financ Econ 81:215–225
9. Korteweg AG (2010) The net benefits to leverage. J Financ 65:2137–2170
10. Van Binsbergen JH, Graham JR, Jie Y (2010) The cost of debt. J Financ 65(6):2089–2136
11. Andrade G, Kaplan SN (1998) How costly is financial (not economic) distress? evidence from highly levered transactions that became distressed. J Financ 53:1443–1493
12. Chen H (2010) Macroeconomic conditions and the puzzles of credit spreads and capital structure. J Financ 65:2171–2212
13. Ju N, Parrino R, Poteshman A, Iisbach M (2005) Horses and rabbits? Trade-off theory and optimal capital structure. J Financ Quant Anal 40:259–282
14. Graya DF, Merton R, Bodiec Z (2007) Contingent claims approach to measuring and managing sovereign credit risk. J Invest Manage 5(4):5–28
15. Leland HE, Toft K (1996) Optimal capital structure, endogenous bankruptcy, and the term structure of credit spreads. J Financ 51:987–1019
16. Stohs MH, Mauer DC (1996) The determinants of corporate debt maturity structure. J Bus 69:279–312
17. Ross SA, Westerfield RW, Jaffe J (2005) Corporate finance (Chapter 16). The McGraw Hill Companies Inc., New York
18. Brealey RA, Myers SC (2003) Principles of corporate finance (Chapter 18). The McGraw Hill Companies Inc., New York
19. Servaes H, Tufano P (2006) The theory and practice of corporate capital structure, deutsche bank. Global survey of corporate financial policies & practices
20. Leary MT, Roberts MR (2005) Do firms rebalance their capital structures? J Financ 60:2575–2619
21. Miller MH (1977) Debt and Taxes. J Financ 32:261–275
22. Graham JR, Harvey C (2001) The theory and practice of corporate finance: evidence from the field. J Financ Econ 60:187–243
23. Tserlukevich Y (2008) Can real options explain financing behavior? J Financ Econ 89:232–252
24. Bradley M, Jarrell G, Kim E (1984) On the existence of an optimal capital structure: theory and evidence. J Financ 39:857–877
25. Strebulaev IA (2007) Do tests of capital structure theory mean what they say? J Financ 62:1747–1787

26. Myers SC, Majluf N (1984) Corporate financing and investment decisions when firms have information that investors do not have. J Financ Econ 13:187–222
27. Baker M, Wurgler J (2002) Market timing and capital structure. J Financ 57:1–32
28. Brennan MJ, Schwartz ES (1984) Optimal financial policy and firm valuation. J Financ 39:593–607
29. Fischer E, Heinkel R, Zechner J (1989) Dynamic capital structure choice: Theory and tests. J Financ 44:19–40
30. Goldstein RS, Ju N, Leland H (2001) An EBIT-based model of dynamic capital structure. J Bus 74:483–512

Printed by Printforce, the Netherlands